A military dictionary. Explaining all difficult terms in martial discipline, fortification, and gunnery. The third edition, improv'd. To which is likewise added, a sea-dictionary of all the terms of navigation

A military dictionary. Explaining all difficult terms in martial discipline, fortification, and gunnery. The third edition, improv'd. To which is likewise added, a sea-dictionary of all the terms of navigation. ... By officers who serv'd several years at
Multiple Contributors, See Notes
ESTCID: T138011
Reproduction from British Library
The first edition of 1702 is anonymous; succeeding editions with varying attributions of authorship.
London : printed; and sold by J. Morphew, 1708.
[312]p.,plate ; 12°

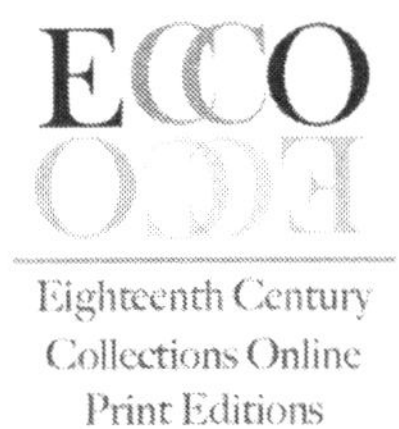

Gale ECCO Print Editions

Relive history with *Eighteenth Century Collections Online*, now available in print for the independent historian and collector. This series includes the most significant English-language and foreign-language works printed in Great Britain during the eighteenth century, and is organized in seven different subject areas including literature and language; medicine, science, and technology; and religion and philosophy. The collection also includes thousands of important works from the Americas.

The eighteenth century has been called "The Age of Enlightenment." It was a period of rapid advance in print culture and publishing, in world exploration, and in the rapid growth of science and technology – all of which had a profound impact on the political and cultural landscape. At the end of the century the American Revolution, French Revolution and Industrial Revolution, perhaps three of the most significant events in modern history, set in motion developments that eventually dominated world political, economic, and social life.

In a groundbreaking effort, Gale initiated a revolution of its own: digitization of epic proportions to preserve these invaluable works in the largest online archive of its kind. Contributions from major world libraries constitute over 175,000 original printed works. Scanned images of the actual pages, rather than transcriptions, recreate the works ***as they first appeared.***

Now for the first time, these high-quality digital scans of original works are available via print-on-demand, making them readily accessible to libraries, students, independent scholars, and readers of all ages.

For our initial release we have created seven robust collections to form one the world's most comprehensive catalogs of 18th century works.

Initial Gale ECCO Print Editions collections include:

> ***History and Geography***
> Rich in titles on English life and social history, this collection spans the world as it was known to eighteenth-century historians and explorers. Titles include a wealth of travel accounts and diaries, histories of nations from throughout the world, and maps and charts of a world that was still being discovered. Students of the War of American Independence will find fascinating accounts from the British side of conflict.

Social Science

Delve into what it was like to live during the eighteenth century by reading the first-hand accounts of everyday people, including city dwellers and farmers, businessmen and bankers, artisans and merchants, artists and their patrons, politicians and their constituents. Original texts make the American, French, and Industrial revolutions vividly contemporary.

Medicine, Science and Technology

Medical theory and practice of the 1700s developed rapidly, as is evidenced by the extensive collection, which includes descriptions of diseases, their conditions, and treatments. Books on science and technology, agriculture, military technology, natural philosophy, even cookbooks, are all contained here.

Literature and Language

Western literary study flows out of eighteenth-century works by Alexander Pope, Daniel Defoe, Henry Fielding, Frances Burney, Denis Diderot, Johann Gottfried Herder, Johann Wolfgang von Goethe, and others. Experience the birth of the modern novel, or compare the development of language using dictionaries and grammar discourses.

Religion and Philosophy

The Age of Enlightenment profoundly enriched religious and philosophical understanding and continues to influence present-day thinking. Works collected here include masterpieces by David Hume, Immanuel Kant, and Jean-Jacques Rousseau, as well as religious sermons and moral debates on the issues of the day, such as the slave trade. The Age of Reason saw conflict between Protestantism and Catholicism transformed into one between faith and logic -- a debate that continues in the twenty-first century.

Law and Reference

This collection reveals the history of English common law and Empire law in a vastly changing world of British expansion. Dominating the legal field is the *Commentaries of the Law of England* by Sir William Blackstone, which first appeared in 1765. Reference works such as almanacs and catalogues continue to educate us by revealing the day-to-day workings of society.

Fine Arts

The eighteenth-century fascination with Greek and Roman antiquity followed the systematic excavation of the ruins at Pompeii and Herculaneum in southern Italy; and after 1750 a neoclassical style dominated all artistic fields. The titles here trace developments in mostly English-language works on painting, sculpture, architecture, music, theater, and other disciplines. Instructional works on musical instruments, catalogs of art objects, comic operas, and more are also included.

A Generall VIEW and DESCRIPTION of the several Parts of FORTIFICATION.

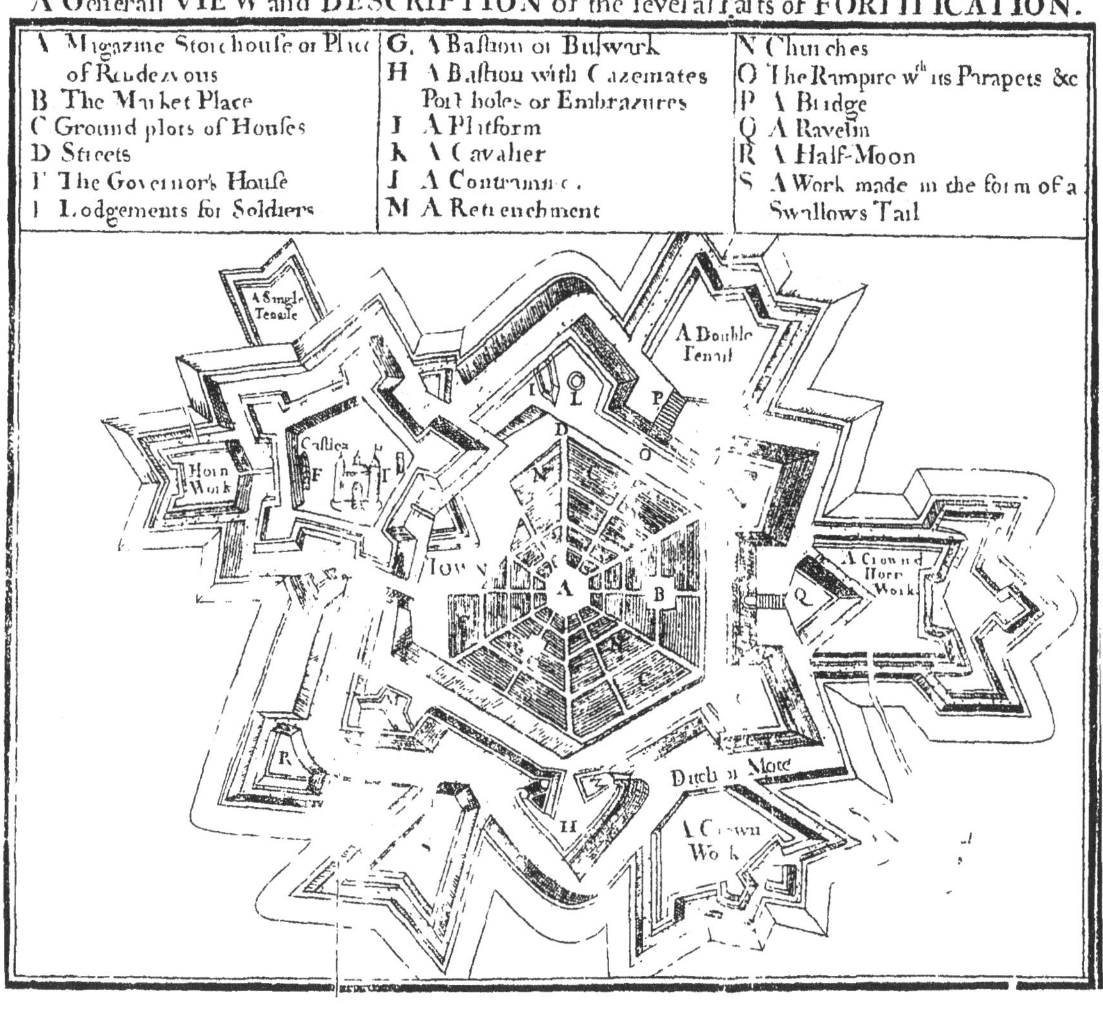

A Military DICTIONARY.

EXPLAINING

All Difficult TERMS in *Martial Discipline*, *Fortification*, and *Gunnery*.

The Third Edition, Improv'd.

To which is likewise added, a

Sea-Dictionary

Of all the Terms of

NAVIGATION.

Both of them very useful (to all Persons that read the Publick News, or serve in the Army, Navy, or Militia) for the Understanding the Accounts of *Sieges*, *Battels*, and other Warlike and Marine *Expeditions*, which daily occur in this Time of Action.

By Officers who serv'd several Years at Sea and Land.

LONDON.

Printed, and Sold by *J. Morphew* near *Stationers-Hall*. MDCCVIII.

(Price 1 *s.* 6 *d.*)

TO THE
READER.

EVery Art and Science has its peculiar Terms, which are obscure to all who are not vers'd in it, or at least have not made it their Business to be acquainted with them. The Art of War, like all the rest, has many Words unknown, or at least not familiar to any but those whose Profession and Duty obliges to be Masters of them. Yet there are but few Men who do not eagerly hearken after, or read News; and at this Time, when all Europe *is embroil'd in War, there can be little News without some Account of Martial Exploits, where there always occur some Terms of Art, not intelligible to Persons unskill'd in Military Affairs. These Difficulties are generally pass'd by unregarded, as if not material for*

 the

the Understanding of what is read; and yet in Reality they are as necessary and proper to be known as any other Part of the Relation, which, without them, becomes but a confus'd Notion of something done or acted, without any distinct judicious Knowledge of the Methods, Parts, and Circumstances of the Action. This little Dictionary *will clear all those Difficulties that may arise from such Terms of Art as are not commonly known; for here they are all Explain'd, not in obscure Words, as if they were design'd for Artists only, but in such a plain familiar Method, as may render them easy to all Capacities. If it happen, as it often does, that one Term is explain'd by another not known to the Reader, he need only turn to it, and thus at one View become Master of them both, for to explain every Word in every Place it is mention'd, would have made a much bigger Book, without any Advantage to the Buyer, who will here find every Word in its proper Place; and the whole* Dictionary *no Burden to his Pocket.*

The

To the Reader.

The same that is said in Behalf of the Military, *answers the End of the* Sea-Dictionary. *The Maritime Terms here explain'd, are not commonly known and intelligible to Land-Men, who, if any Thing Curious, must be well pleas'd to understand them, as they occur in Relations, which cannot possibly be without them.*

The Method here follow'd is plain and easy, adapted to every Capacity; so that this little Pocket-Book may be of Use to all Men. The Soldier may learn the Language of the Sea, and the Sailor that of the Army. The less Learned will be so instructed, so as to speak properly to both; and the able Scholar will find that Sort of Information, which is not to be met with in great Libraries. In short, at this Time nothing seems to be more necessary for all Sorts of Persons; and what is more, the Bulk is such as renders it Portable with Ease, and the Price so inconsiderable, that no Exception can be made against it.

Advertisements.

THE *Art of WAR* In 4 Parts. Containing, 1 The Duties of Officers of Horse 2 Of Officers of Foot 3 Of a Soldier in general; with Variety of Examples of such as have been disgrac'd for being ignorant of them 4 The Rules and Practices of War by all great Generals; the Order of Marching, Encamping, Fighting, Attacking and Defending strong Places; and the Method of surprizing Garisons or Armies, and of beating up of Quarters. Written in *French* by Four able Officers of long Service and Experience; and Translated into *English* by an *English* Officer Illustrated with several Cuts The Second Edition. Sold by *J Morphew* near *Stationers-Hall*

LIVES, English and Foreign, viz *William* Lord *Burleigh*, Sir *Water Raleigh*, *George* Duke of *Buckingham*, Marquiss of *Montross*, *Oliver Cromwell*, Admiral *Coligni*, Don *John* of *Austria*, *William* the First Prince of *Orange*, *Alexander Farnese* Prince of *Parma*, *Albert* Count *Wallenstein*, Duke of *Hamilton*, General *Blake*, Duke of *Albemarle*, Earl of *Shaftsbury*, Duke of *Monmouth*, Admiral *Ruyter*, Viscount *Turenne*, Prince of *Conde*, Admiral *Tromp*, Duke and of *Lorrain.* These Lives contain the History of our own and other Nations, from the Year 1550, to the Year 1690. By several Hands: Who have been assisted in the Work with many private Memoirs. In Two Volumes in *8vo* Printed for *B Tooke* at the *Middle-Temple* Gate in *Fleet-street*; and sold by *J Morphew* near *Stationers-Hall* Price 12 *s*

The Present State of the Universe; or, An Account of, 1. The Rise, Births, Names, Matches, Children, and near Allies, of all the present Chief Princes of the World 2 Their Coats of Arms, Motto's, Devices, Liveries, Religions, and Languages. 3 The Names of their Chief Towns, with some Computation of the Houses and Inhabitants: Their Chief Seats of Pleasure, and other remarkable Things in their Dominions. 4. Their Revenues, Power and Strength. 5 Their respective Styles and Titles, or Apellations 6 And an Account of the Commonwealths, relating to the same Heads To this Fourth Edition, continued and enlarg'd, with several Effigies wanting in the former Impression; as also the various Bearings of their several Ships at Sea; are added their several Territories, which are distant from them in other Parts of the World. 12°. Sold by *J. Morphew* near *Stationers-Hall*

The History of Queen Anne's *Reign* Digested into Annals. In Six Volumes. Printed for *A Roper* at the *Black-Boy* over against St. *Dunstan's* Church in *Fleet-street*.

A
Military Dictionary.

A.

A*Djutant* Vide *Aid-Major*
Advanc'd Guard Vide *Guard*
Aid de Camp An Officer always following one of the Generals, hat is, the General, Lieutenant-General, r Major-General, to receive and carry heir Orders, as occasion requires When he King is in the Field, he appoints oung Gentlemen of Note to carry his Orders, and they are call'd the King's *Aids de Camp*
Advance To advance, is to move forwards *Advance your Pikes*, is to hold them upight close to the Right Side, the But-End n the Right Hand
Aid Major, or *Adjutant*. An Officer who eases the Major of part of the Burhen of his Duty, and performs it all in is Absence Some Majors have several *Aids-Majors* Each Troop of Guards has ut one Major, who has two *Aids-Majors* very fortify'd Place has but one Major, who has more or fewer *Aids-Majors* uner him, according to its bigness. Every egiment of Foot has as many *Aids-Ma-*

jors as it contains Battalions When a Battalion is drawn up, the *Aid-Major's* Post is on the Left, beyond all the Captains, and behind the Lieutenant-Colonel.

Alarm By some falsely writ *Alarum* is a sudden Apprehension upon some Noise or Report, which makes Men run to their Arms to stand upon their Guard There are false Alarms, when they are taken upon false Fears or Reports, or else when given by the Enemy, only to keep their Adversaries from rest, or otherwise to deceive them

Ambuscade, or *Ambush* A Body of Men that lies conceal'd in a Wood, or other convenient Place, to surprise or enclose an Enemy To fall into an Ambush, to discover an Ambush, to defeat an Ambush

Ambligon Vide *Triangle*.

Ammunition, implies all sorts of Warlike Stores, and more particularly Powder and Ball

Ammunition Bread The Bread that is provided for, and distributed to the Soldiers.

Angle, as a Geometrical Term in general, is the meeting of Two Lines, and touching one another in the same Plain, yet not lying in the same straight Line, but so that, if prolong'd, they would cut one another, and so form another Angle upon the Back of the first.

An

A N

An Acute Angle That which is sharp and less open than the Right Angle, in measure under 90 Degrees

An Obtuse Angle That which is blunt, and more open than a Right Angle, in measure above 90 Degrees

An Angle Rectilinear, is made by straight Lines, to distinguish it from the Spherical or Curvilinear, of which no more need be said, as being of no use in Fortification

A Right Angle, is form'd by a Line falling perpendicularly upon another, and the measure of this Angle is always 90 Degrees

Angle at the Center, in Fortification, is that which is form'd in the midst of the *Polygon*, or Figure, by two Lines proceeding from the Center, and terminating at the two nearest Angles of the Polygon

Angle of the Curtin, or *Angle of the Flank* That which is made by and contain'd between the Curtin and the Flank, as *H I L* *Fig* 1

Angle of the Polygon That which is made by the meeting of the two sides of the *Polygon*, or Figure, in the Center of the Bastion

Angle of the Triangle Half the Angle of the *Polygon*

Angle of the Bastion, or *Flank'd Angle* That which is made by the two Faces, being the utmost part of the Bastion, most expos'd to the Enemies Batteries and called the Point of the Bastion.

Angle diminiſh'd Only us'd by the Dutch Engineers, and compos'd by the Face of the Baſtion, and the exterior Side of the Polygon.

Angle of the Shoulder, or *Epaule* Form'd by the Face and Flank of the Baſtion

Angle at the Flank Vide *Angle at the Curtin*

Angle of the Tenaille, or outward *Flanking Angle*, call'd alſo *Angle Mort*, or *Dead Angle*, or *Angle Rentrant*, or *Angle Inwards* Made by the two Lines *Fichant*, that is, the Faces of the two Baſtions extended till they meet in an Angle towards the Curtin, and is that which always carries its Point in towards the Work

Angle forming the Flank Made by the Flank, and that part of the Side of the *Polygon* which runs from the ſaid Flank to the Angle of the *Polygon*, and if protracted croſſes the Baſtion, only us'd by Dutch Engineers

Flank'd Angle The Angle made by the two Faces of the Baſtion, the Point of the Baſtion

Angle Saillant, *Sortant*, or *Viff*. That which thruſts out its Point from the Work towards the Country.

Angle Rentrant An Angle pointing inwards, as the *Saillant* does outwards

Inward-Flanking Angle. That which is made by the Flanking Line, and the Curtin.

Ang

Angle of the Counterscarp Made by two Sides of the Counterscarp before the middle of the Curtin

Angles of a Battalion Made by the last Men at the ends of the Ranks and Files

Front-Angles The two last Men of the Front-Rank

Rear-Angles The two last Men of the Rear-Rank

Anspesade Vide *Lanspesade*

Antestature A small Retrenchment made with Palisades, or Bags of Earth, wherewith Men cover themselves in haste, to dispute the rest of the Ground when the Enemy has gain'd part

Appointé A Foot Soldier, who for his long Service, and extraordinary Bravery, receives pay above the private Sentinels, and expects to be advanc'd This is in *France*, for I find none such in *England*; and now even in *France* the *Appointees* of all Regiments have been suppress'd, since the Companies are reduc'd to 50 Men, Only the Regiment of Guards has still 40 *Appointees* in a Company, each Company consisting of 150 Men Their extraordinary Allowance is 18 Deniers above the other Soldiers

Approaches All the Works that are carry'd on towards a Place that is Besieg'd; as the Trenches, Epaulments without Trenches, Redoubts Places of Arms, Sappe, Galeries, and Lodgments *See these Words in their several Places* Approaches *also signify* Attacks

Araignée, Rameau, Branch, Return o Galery of a Mine Vide *Galery*

Area The Superficial Content of an Rampart, or other Works, in solid Feet o Earth

Army A numerous Body of Troops consisting of Horse, Foot and Dragoons commanded by a General

Flying Army Vide *Camp*

Arsenal A Place appointed for making and keeping of all Warlike Stores

Artillery All sorts of Great Guns, Mortars, Petards, and the like The Trai of Artillery, includes all sorts of Warlike Stores There is a General, Comptroller, and very many other Offices belonging to the Artillery, too long for this Place Vide *Cannon*

Assault The Effort Men make, and the Fight they engage in, to make themselves Masters of a Post, and gain it by main force, driving the Defendants from it and exposing their Bodies to this Purpose to the Fire of the Besieged, without the Defence of any Works. Whilst the Assault lasts, and both Parties are mix'd there is no Danger of the Cannon on either Side, because both are afraid of destroying their own Men among the Enemies To give an Assault, To be commanded to the Assault; To stand an Assault, To second the Assault To repulse an Assault; To carry the Assault

To Assault Vide *to Insult*

Attack The General Assault, or Onset, that is given to gain a Post, or upon any Body of Troops

Attack of a Siege. The Works the Besiegers carry on, either Trenches, Galleries, Sapps or Breaches, to reduce a Place on any of its Sides Sometimes two Attacks are carried on against one same *Tenaille*, or Front of a Place, with Lines of Communication between them *Vide* Trenches

False Attack That which is not carry'd on with such Vigour as the rest, as not intended to do the same Effect, but only to give a Diversion to the Besieged, and divide the Garison, and yet sometimes the false Attack has prov'd as successful as the Real

Regular or *Droit Attacks* Those which are carry'd on in Form, according to Rules of Art

Avant-Fosse, or Ditch of the Counterscarp A Moat or Ditch full of Water running round the Counterscarp, on the outside next the Campaign, at the Foot of the Glacis. Engineers do not approve of it, where there is a Possibility of dreining it, because then it is a Trench ready made for the Besiegers to defend themselves against the Sallies of the Besieged; and besides, it obstructs the putting of Succours into the Place, or at least makes it more difficult

B

BAGS vide *Canvas Bags*

Ball Vide *Bullet* and *Fireball*

Ban A Proclamation made at the Head of a Body of Troops, or in the several Quarters of the Army, by Sound of Trumpet, or Beat of Kettle-Drums or Drums, either for observing of Martial Discipline, or for declaring a new Officer, or punishing a Soldier, or the like

Bandaleers Little wooden Cases cover'd with Leather, of which every Musketeer wears 12 hanging on a Shoulder-Belt, or Collar, as they call it, each of them contains the Charge of Powder for a Musket

Bands Bodies of Foot properly, as the *French* formerly call'd all their Infantry, *Bands Françoises*, or *French* Bands but not now us'd In *England*, the Word is still us'd for the Band of Pensioners a Company of Gentlemen attending the King's Person upon Solemn Occasions

Banquette Vide *Footbank*

Barack, or *Baraque* A Hut, like a little Cottage, for Soldiers to lie in the Camp Once only those of the Horse were call'd Baracks, and those of the Foot Huts, but now the Name is indifferently given to both These are made, either when the Soldiers have not Tents

Tents, or when any Army lies long in a Place in bad Weather, because they keep out Cold, Heat or Rain, better than Tents, and are otherwise more commodious They are generally made, by fixing four strong forked Poles in the Ground, and laying four others a-cross them, then they build the Walls with Wattles or Sods, or such as the Place affords The Top is either Thatch'd, if there be Straw to spare, or covered with Planks, or sometimes with Turf

Barbe To fire *en Barbe*, is to fire the Cannon over the Parapet, instead of putting it through *Embrazures* To fire thus, the Parapet must be but three Foot and a half high

Barm, or *Berm* Vide *Foreland*

Barricado A Fence made of Palisades.

Barril of a Gun, or Pistol. Is all the Iron Cavity into which the Powder and Ball are convey'd, the great Length beyond that which is so filled, serving to give the great Strength to the Shot by its longer Confinement

Barrils These fill'd with Earth, serve to make Parapets to cover the Men, like the Gabions and Canvas-Bags

Base The Level Line on which any Work stands, that is even with the Ground or Campaign.

A Base The smallest Piece of Cannon, that is, carrying a Ball but of 5 Ounces.

Base-Ring of a Cannon. The great Ring next to and behind the Touch-hole

Baskets or *Corbeilles* Are uſed to b fill'd with Earth, and placed one by another, to cover the Men from the Enemies Shot They are wider at the Top than at the Bottom, that there may be ſpace enough below for the Men to fire thro' upon the Enemy They are generally a Foot, or a Foot and half high

Baſſe-Enceinte, or *Baſſe-Encloſure* The ſame as *Fauſſe Braye*

Baſtion A great Work ſometimes fac'd or lin'd with Stone or Brick, and ſometimes with Sods, generally advancing before an Angle of the *Polygon* towards the Campaign The Lines terminating it, are Two Faces, Two Flanks, and Two Demigorges, The Union of the Two Faces makes the outmoſt Angle, call'd the *Angle of the Baſtion* The Union of the Two Faces to the Two Flanks, makes the Side Angles called the *Shoulders* or *Epauls*, and the Union of the two other Ends of the Flanks to the two Curtins, forms the Angles of the Flanks

A Baſtion compos'd Is when the two Sides of the Interior *Polygon* are very unequal, which makes the *Gorges* alſo unequal

A Baſtion cut off with a Tenaille, in French *Baſtion coupé*, or *Baſtion a Tenaille* Is that whoſe Point is cut off, and makes an Angle inwards, and two Points outwards, that is a *Tenaille*. This is done when Water, or any other Accident, hinders carrying on the Baſtion to its full Extent, or that it would be too ſhort.

A Baſtion

A Bastion deform'd That which wants one of the Demigorges, because one Side of the Interior *Polygon* is so very short

A Demi-Bastion, has but one Face and Flank, and is usually before a Horn-work, or Crown-work It is also called an *Epaulment*

A Bastion detach'd, or *cut off* That which is separated from the Body of the Works

A Double Bastion That which is on the Plain of the great Bastion, has another Bastion built higher, leaving 12 or 18 Feet between the Parapet of the lower, and the Foot of the higher

A hollow or *voided Bastion*, in French, *Bastion Vuide*, or *Creux* Has only a Rampart and Parapet about its Flanks and Faces, leaving an empty Space towards the Center, and the Earth so low, that when an Enemy is once lodg'd on the Rampart, there is no making a Retrenchment towards the Center, but what will be under the Fire of the Besiegers

A Plat Bastion If the Distance between the Angles of the Interior *Polygon* be double the usual Length, then a Bastion is made in the middle before the Curtin or straight Line, whereas the others are generally before the Angles, and this is call'd a *Plat-Bastion* It has generally this Disadvantage attending it: That unless there be an extraordinary Breadth

allow'd

allow'd to the Moat, the returning Angle of the Counterscarp runs back too far into the Ditch, and hinders the Sight and Defence of the two opposite Flanks

A Regular Bastion Is that which has a due Proportion of Faces, Flanks and Gorges

A Solid Bastion, rises equally to the Rampaits of the Place, without any empty Space towards the Center They have this Advantage above others, that they afford Earth enough to make a Retrenchment in case the Enemy lodge himself on the Top of the Bastion, and the Besieged are resolved to dispute every Foot of Ground

Battalion A Body of Foot commonly consisting of 7 or 800 Men, Two Thirds whereof are generally Musketeers, and the other Third Pikemen, who are posted in the Center *Battalions* are for the most part drawn up Six deep, that is, Six Men in File, or one before another, those in Length, or Side by Side, being call'd *Ranks* Some Regiments consist of but one Battalion, but if more numerous they are divided into several Battalions, according to their Strength, so that every one may be about the Number aforesaid So the Battalions of *French* Guards have commonly but 5 Companies, because each of those Companies have 150 Men, but of other *French* Regiments, there go 16 Companies to make

make up a Battalion, because they are but 50 Men in a Company Of the *Swisse* Guards, Four Companies make a Battalion, because they are 180 in a Company When there are Companies of several Regiments in a Garison, and they are to form a Battalion, those of the Eldest Regiment post themselves on the Right, those of the Second on the Left, and so the others successively on the Right and Left, till the Youngest fall into the Center The Subaltern Officers take their Posts before their Companies, the Captains on the Right and Left according to their Degree Battalions are divided into Three great Divisions, which are the Musketeers on the Right and Left, and the Pikes in the Center In marching, when there is not room for so large a Front, they break into Sub divisions, according as the Ground will allow The Art of drawing up Battalions, teaches how to range a Body of Foot in such Order and Form, that it may most advantageously engage a greater Body, either of Horse and Foot, or both, but the main Design is to prevent the Foot being broke by the Horse, when attack'd in open Field, where there are no Ditches, Hedges, or other Advantages, to secure them Formerly they used to reduce the Battalion to an *Octogon*, or Figure of 8 Sides, and since the hollow Square has been us'd; but both these Methods require

quire too much Time upon ſudden Oc-
caſions, and Men muſt be very well
diſciplin'd, or it will put them in-
greater Confuſion

Battery or *Platform* A Place to plant Guns on It is laid with Planks and Sleepers for them to reſt on, that the Wheels of the Carriages may not ſink into the Earth They are allow'd a little Stoop, or inclining towards the Parapet, that the Guns may recoil the leſs, and be more eaſily return'd to their Place Field or Camp Batteries are to have a Ditch before them, to be Paliſado'd, and have a Parapet on them, and two Redoubts on the Flanks, or Places of Arms, to cover the Troops that are to defend them The open Spaces in the Parapet, to put the Muzzles of the Guns out at, are call'd *Embrazures*, and the Diſtances between the Embrazures, *Merlons*. The Guns are generally about 12 Foot diſtant from one another, that the Parapet may be ſtrong, and the Gunners have room to work

Battery ſunk, or *bury'd* In French, *Batterie Enterre*, or *Ruinante*. When the Platform is ſunk into the Ground, ſo that there muſt be Trenches cut in the Earth againſt the Muzzles of the Guns for them to fire out at, or to ſerve as Embrazures This ſort of Battery is generally us'd upon firſt making the Approaches to beat down the Parapet of the Place.

Ca-

Cross Batteries. Two Batteries which play athwart one another upon the same Body, forming an Angle there, and beat with more Violence, whence follows more Destruction, because what one Bullet shakes, the other beats down

Battery d'Enfilade That which scours or sweeps the whole Length of a straight Line

Battery en Echarp That which plays on any Work obliquely

Battery de Revers, or *Murdering Battery* That which beats upon the Back

Joint Battery, or *Batterie par Camarade* When several Guns fire at the same time upon one Body To raise a Battery to plant a Battery, to ruin a Battery

Batterie de Tambour The *French* so called the Beat of Drum, which we call the General *Vide* General, to beat the General

Batteurs d'Estrade Scouts or Discoverers, Horsemen sent out before and on the Wings of an Army, a Mile, Two or Three, to discover, and give the General Account of what they see.

Battle The Engagement of Two Armies

Battle Array The Order of Battle; the Form of Drawing up the Army for Fight

Main Battle In French, *Corps de Bataille.* The main Body of the Army, which is the Second of the Two Lines, whereof the First is the Van, and the

Third

Third the Rear, or Reserve *Vide* Line

Bayonette A Broad Dagger without any Guard, generally made with a round taper Handle to stick it in the Muzzle of a Musket, in which manner it serves instead of a Pike to receive the Charge of Horse, all the Men having first the Advantage of their Shot, and then as many as there is occasion for, with their Bayonets thus in their Muskets, cover the rest of the Musketeers

To Beat a Parley Vide *Chamade* For this, and all other Beats, *vide* Drum

Beetles Great Sledges, or Hammers to drive down Palisades, or for other Uses.

Berme Vide *Foreland*

Biovac A Guard at Night perform'd by the whole Army, which either at a Siege, or lying before an Enemy, every Evening draws out from its Tents or Huts, and continues all Night under Arms before its Lines or Camp, to prevent any Surprise When Troops are much harass'd, or there is no great Apprehension of the Enemy, sometimes it is allowed the *Biovac*, that the two Front Ranks by Turns stand under Arms, whilst the Rear Ranks take some Rest on the Ground The Word *Biovac*, is a Corruption of the *German Weinack*, which signifies Double Guard To raise the *Biovac*, is to return the Army to their Tents or Huts some time after break of Day

Blinds

Blindes Pieces of Wood to lay a croſs a Trench, to bear the Faſcine, or Clays laid on them loaded with Earth, to cover the Workmen This is generally done when the Work is about the Glacis, and the Trench is carry'd on facing the Place.

Blindes are alſo ſometimes only Canvas ſtretch'd to take away the ſight of the Enemy, ſometimes they are Planks ſet up, for which *ſee* Mantelets, others of Baskets, for which *ſee* Gabions, others of Barrils, and others of Sacks fill'd with Earth But moſt properly Blindes are Bundles of Oziers, or other ſmall Wood bound at both Ends, and ſet up between Stakes or Clays

Blind, is alſo the ſame as *Orillon*

Bloccade, or *Blocus*. Is in the Nature of a Siege, when Troops are poſted on all the Avenues that lead to the Place, in order to keep out any Supplies from going into it; ſo that it is propos'd to ſtarve it out, and not take it by Regular Attacks To form a Bloccade, to raiſe a Bloccade, to turn a Siege into a Bloccade

To Bloccade, or *Block up a Place* To ſhut up all the Avenues, ſo that it can receive no Relief

Blunderbuſs A ſhort Fire-Arm with a very large Bore to carry a Number of Musket or Piſtol Bullets, proper to do Execution in a Crowd, or to make good a narrow Paſſage, as the Door of a Houſe, Stair-Caſe, or the like

Bomb

Bomb An Iron Shell, or hollow Ball with a large Touch-hole to put in a *Fuz* which is made of a Composition that is to burn slowly, that it may last all the time the Bomb is flying, and the Fu not come to the Powder within till it falls, and so do Execution by firing wh is about it, or by the Pieces of the Shell flying about This Bomb is clapp'd int a Mortar-piece mounted on a Carriage and when the Bombardier has set Fire to the Fuzé with one hand, he gives Fire to the Touch-hole of the Mortar-piece with the other. Bombs may be us'd without Mortar-pieces, as the *Venetians* did at *Candia*, when the *Turks* had pos sessed themselves of the Ditch, rolling down Bombs upon them along a Plank set stooping towards their Works, with Ledges on the Sides to keep the Bom right forwards They are also bury'd under Ground to blow it up, for which see *Caisson*

Bonnet A Work consisting of two Faces, which make an Angle Saillant in the Nature of a small Ravelin, without any Ditch, having only a Parapet, thre Foot high, and Palisado'd, with anothe Palisade at 10 or 12 Foot distance The *Bonnet* is made beyond the Counterscarp in the Nature of a little advanc'd *Corps de Garde*

Bonnet a' Prestre, or *Priests Cap* An Out work, which at the Head has three An gles Saillant, and two inwards, an

diff

differs from the double *Tenaille* only in this Point That its Sides, instead of being Parallel, are made like the *Queve d'Yronde*, or Swallow's Tail, that is, narrowing or drawing close at the Gorge, and opening at the Head

Boyau, or *Branch of the Trenches* A Line or particular Cut that runs from the Trenches to cover some Spot of Ground, and is drawn Parallel to the Works of the Place, that it may not be enfiladed, that is, that the Shot from the Town may not scour along it Sometimes a *Boyau* is a Line of Communication from one Trench to another, when two Attacks are carried on near one another. Their Parapet being always next to the Place besieg'd, they do the Service of a Line of Contravallation, to hinder Sallies, and cover the Pioneers.

Branch· As *Boyau* above.

Branch of a Mine Vide *Galery*

Breach The Ruin of any Part of the Works beaten down with Cannon, or blown up by Mine, to make it fit to give an Assault To make good the Breach; to fortify the Breach with *Chevaux de Frize*, to make a Lodgment on the Breach; to clear the Breach, that is, to remove the Ruins, that it may be the better defended

To Break Ground To begin the Works for carrying on the Siege about a Town, or Fort.

Breast-

Breast-work Vide *Parapet*

Breech of a Gun Is the strongest Part of it behind the Place where the Charge lies, being solid and strong to bear the Recoil of the Powder

Brigade A Party or Body, either of Horse or Foot, for there are Two sorts of Brigades, *viz* A Brigade of an Army, and a Brigade of a Troop of Horse A Brigade of an Army is either of Horse or Foot, and not fix'd of what Number or Force it must be, for the Brigade of Horse may consist of Eight, Ten or Twelve Squadrons, and that of Foot of Three, Four, Five, or Six Battalions The Brigade of a Troop of Horse is the Third part of it, when it does not exceed 40 or 50 Men, but if the Troops be 100 strong, it is divided into Six Brigades The Troops of Horse-Guards are divided into Brigades.

Brigadier The Officer that commands a Brigade Brigadiers of the Army, are those that command a Brigade of so many Squadrons of Horse, or Battalions of Foot, as was mentioned speaking of the Brigade of an Army, they having the Fourth Degree in the Army, as being next in Command to the Major-Generals Every Brigadier marches at the Head of his Brigade upon Service The Brigadier of Foot commands him of Horse in Garison; and the Brigadier of Horse him of Foot in the Field Brigadiers of the Horse-Guards comman[d] is youngest Captains of Horse Other Troops of Horse in *France* have Brigadiers, which they have not in *England*, where they are called Corporals of Horse

Bridge The Word in general needs no Exposition, but this may be said in relation to it, That of late Years Copper Boats have been much us'd to be carry'd in Armies for laying Bridges over Rivers upon occasion, which is done by joyning these Boats side by side, till they reach a-cross the River, and laying Planks over them to make all plain for the Men to march upon

Flying Bridge, or *Pont Volant* Is made of two small Bridges laid one over the other, in such manner that the uppermost stretches and runs out, by the help of certain Cords running through Pulleys placed along the Sides of the Under-Bridge, which push it forwards, till the End of it joyns the Place it is designed to be fix'd on When these two Bridges are stretch'd out at their full Length, so that the two middle Ends meet, they must not be above Four or Five Fathom long, because if longer they will break; and therefore they are only us'd to surprize Out-works, or Posts, that have but narrow Moats Flying-Bridges are also us'd to be carry'd upon Rivers, but they are only great Boats with Planks, and all necessarily to joyn, and make a Bridge in a very short time, as occasion requires

Bridge of Rushes, or *Pont de Jonc* A Bridge made of great Bundles of Rushes that grow in marshy Grounds, which being bound together, have Planks fastned on them, and are so laid over Morasses or Boggy Places for the Horse and Foot to march over They have also been us'd to pass the Moat of a Place besieged, and are not so easy to be burnt as Fascines, tho' these be loaded with Earth

Draw-Bridge A Bridge made fast only at one End with Hinges, so that the other End may be lifted up, and then the Bridge stands upright to hinder the Passage of the Moat There are others made to draw back to hinder the Passage, and to thrust over again to pass Again, there are others which open in the Middle, and one half of them turns away to one Side, and the other to the other Side, and so are joyned again at Pleasure, but these are not so proper, because one half of them remains on the Enemy's Side

Bringers up The whole last Rank of a Battalion drawn up, being the hindmost Men of every File.

Bullet, *Ball*, or *Shot* The Ball of Iron or Lead that is fired out of a Cannon, Musket, or Pistol, for it comprehends all Sorts That of the whole Cannon weighs 48 Pounds, of the Bastard-Cannon 42, of the Ordinary Demi-Cannon 32, the Twenty four Pounder 24 of the la[rge]

Cul[verin]

ulverin 20, of the Twelve Pounder 12, f the large Demi-Culverin 12, of the x Pounder 6, of the Saker about 5, of e Minion about 4, of the Three Pounder 3, of the Drakes, Pedreroes, and his, gradually less All these are of on The Musket-Ball is about an unce, the Carabine and Pistol less, and ese of Lead Red-hot Bullets are shot Sieges to fire Houses, and do the ore Mischief in a Town They are so ated in a Forge made for the purpose ose by the Battery, whence they are ken out with an Iron Ladle, and rown into the Pieces, into which bere a good Tompion of Sod or Turf ramm'd down, that the Bullet may not uch the Powder

Bulwark The Ancient Name for a stion, now antiquated *Vide* Bastion

C

CAdet A Voluntier that serves upon his own Charge, as young Genemen do, carrying Arms to learn Exrience, and wait for Preferment In *ance*, the King allows but two *Cadets* be received into any one Company Foot. The proper Signification of e Word, is a Younger Brother, and ence apply'd to bear this Sense, beuse Younger Brothers take this upon em to raise their Fortunes.

Caisson,

Caisson, or *Superficial Fourneau* A Wood-en Case or Chest, into which they p[ut] 3 or 4 Bombs, and sometimes to th[e] number of 6, according to the Execu-tion they are to do, or the Ground [is] firmer or looser Sometimes the Che[st] is only fill'd with Powder When th[e] Besieged dispute every Foot of Groun[d] this *Caisson* is bury'd under some Wo[rk] the Enemy intends to possess himself of and when he is Master of it, they [set] fire to it by a Train convey'd in a Pip[e] which blows them up Thus we m[ay] say after the Mine or *Fourneau* had de-stroy'd the *Bonette*, a *Caisson* was bury[d] under the Ground thrown up, and th[e] Enemy advancing to make a Lodgme[nt] on the Ruins of the *Bonette*, the *Caiss[on]* was fir'd, and blew up the Post the Se-cond time

Caisson, is also a Cover'd Waggon [to] carry Bread, or Ammunition

Caliper Compasses Us'd by Gunners [to] measure the Diameter of Bullets, and C[y-]linder of Guns, and therefore the Le[gs] instead of being straight, are made bow[ing] to find the true Diameter of any C[ir-]cle

Calthrops Vide *Crows Feet*

Camp The Ground on which an A[r-]my pitches its Tents, and lodges, som[e-]times intrenching, and sometimes wi[th-]out any other Defence than chusing t[he] Advantage of the Ground.

Flying Camp. A Strong Body of Horse and Foot, commanded for the most part by a Lieutenant General which is always in motion, both to cover its own Garrisons, and to keep the Army in continual Alarm.

Campaign. The time every Year that an Army continues in the Field, during any War. We say, a Man has serv'd so many Campaigns. The Campaign will begin at such a Time. This will be a long Campaign.

Cannon, Orduance, Great Guns, or *Artillery*, Fire Arms, either of Brass or Iron, long, round and hollow, charg'd with Powder and Ball, or Cartridge. There are several Degrees and Sizes of them, distinguish'd by these several Names: Whole Cannon, Bastard Cannon, or Cannon of Seven, Demi-Cannon 24 Pounders, Whole-Culverin 12 Pounders, Demi-Culverin 6 Pounders, Sakers, Minions 3 Pounders, Drakes and Pedreroes; more of each of which, you may see under its proper Letter. Cannon often fir'd must be carefully cool'd, or else it will burst. See more under *Battery, Cavalier, Embrazures*. To Nail, to Recoil, and Carriages.

Cannon Royal, or *of Eight*. A Great Gun, 8 Inches Diameter in the Bore, 12 Foot long, 8000 Pounds Weight, carries a Charge of 32 Pounds of Powder, and a Ball 7 Inches and 4 Eights

 Dia-

Diameter and 48 Pounds Weight. Its point-blank Shot 185 Paces.

Cannon Baskets. Vide *Gabions.*

Canvas Bags, or *Earth Bags.* Are Bags containing about a Cubical Foot of Earth. They are us'd to raise a Parapet in hast, or repair one that is beaten down. These are of use when the Ground is Rocky, and affords not Earth to carry on Approaches, because they can be easily brought from further off, and remov'd at Will. The *French* call them *Sacs-a-Terre*, that is, Earth-Bags. These same Bags, upon occasion, are us'd for Powder, and hold 50 Pounds.

Capital. A Line drawn from the Angle of the *Polygon*, to the Point of the *Bastion*, as C I and D G. *Fig.* 1.

Capitulation. The Conditions on which a Place that is besieg'd surrenders, being Articles agreed between the Besieg'd and Besiegers.

Caponniere. A Work, or Lodgment sunk four or five Foot into the Ground, with its Sides rising about two Foot above the Ground, on which they lay Planks well cover'd with Earth. They are big enough to lodge 15 or 20 Musketeers, who fire through Loop-holes made in the Sides. These are generally made on the Glacis, or in dry Moats.

Captain. The Commander in chief of a Company of Foot, or Troop of Horse or Dragoons. He is to march or fight a

t

the Head of his Company; among the Horse, when Captains of several Regiments meet, he that has the eldest Commission takes Place, and commands; but among the Foot, the Captain of the eldest Regiment commands all that are of younger Regiments, tho' they have elder Commissions

Captain Lieutenant The Commanding Officer of the Colonel's Troop or Company in every Regiment He commands as youngest Captain, tho' in reality he is only Lieutenant, the Colonel being himself Captain In *France*, there are several other Captains-Lieutenants, as those of the two Troops of Musketeers, of Gendarmes, and of the Independent Troops of Light-Horse, whereof the King, Queen, Dauphin, or King's Brother, are Captains Those of the Musketeers, Gendarmes, and Light-Horse, whereof the King himself is Captain takes Place as eldest Colonels of Light Horse, and accordingly command all others The Captains-Lieutenants of the Queens, Dauphin's, and King's Brother's Troops, and the Sub-Lieutenants of the King's Gendarmes, roul with all Colonels of Horse, according to the Dates of their Commissions

Captain en Pied A Captain kept in Pay, that is not reform'd The Expression, tho' altogether *French*, occurs sometimes

Captain Reform'd One, who upon re-ducing of Forces loses his Company, is continu'd Captain, either as Second to another, or without Post *Vide* Re-form'd

Captain en Second Vide *Second*

Captain des Gardes, & aux Gardes Tho' this Distinction be peculiar to *France*, it occurs so often, that it requires to be explain'd. The English of it is Captain of the Guards, or in the Guards *Captain des Gardes*, or Captain of the Guards, is Captain of one of the four Troops of Horse-Guards *Captain aux Gardes*, or Captain in the Guards, is the Captain of a Company in the Regiment of Foot Guards.

Carabine A small Fire-Arm, between a Pistol and a Musket, us'd by all the Horse

Carabineers Some Regiments of chosen Horse cull'd out of all the other Regiments in *France* of late Years

Carcass A mischievous Invention, of the nature of a Bomb, and thrown like it out of a Mortar-piece. It is compos'd of 2, 3, or more Granadoes, and several small Pistol Barrels, charg'd and wrapp'd up with the Granadoes in Towe dipp'd in Oil, and other Combustible Matter The whole is put into a pitch'd Cloth made up Oval, which is set in an Iron Frame like a Lanthorn, having a hollow Top and Bottom, and Bars running between them to hold them together

Th

Theſe long Bars that join the Top and ..ttom, are bound together by one or ..ore Iron Rings, all which in ſome mea..re repreſents the Trunk of a dead Carcaſs One of the Concave Places has .Ring to lift and put it into the Mor..r piece, the other has a Touch-hole to ..t fire to the Carcaſs, which is ſhot ..ke a Bomb upon any Place intended .. be fir'd Theſe Carcaſſes do not an..er as much as was expected from ..em

.. *Caracol*, as *Wheel by Caracol*; us'd on..y among the Horſe, and is a Serpentine ..r Rounding Motion of Wheeling, ſo ..ll'd from the *Spaniſh* Word *Caracol*, a ..nail, becauſe they wind round like that ..reature And *Caracol*, in *Spaniſh*, is ..ence taken for a round or ſpiral Motion.

.. *Carriages* for Guns, are in the nature ..f long narrow Carts, each made to the ..roportion of the Gun it is to carry ..hen they ſtand upon Batteries, they ..ave but two Wheels, and ſo they are ..'d, but when drawn, two other leſs ..heels are added beyond the Breech of ..e Piece The Carriages for Mortars ..e low, with four Wheels each of one ..iece, exactly like the Sea-Carriages

To carry on the Trenches Vide *Trenches*.

.. *Cartridge* In French *Cartouch* A Roll ..f Paper, Paſt-board, or Parchment, like ..Caſe made to contain the Charge of any ..re-Arm Cartridges for Piſtols and

Muskets are made of Paper, which is sufficient to contain that Charge of Powder and Ball, but they are of Past-board or Parchment to hold the Shot, broken Iron, and Powder to charge Cannon when it is to fire near at hand There is this Inconveniency in Musket and Pistol-Cartridges, that they are not easily drawn upon occasion, and besides, they require too much Time for ramming upon hasty firing, but in Cannon or Cazemats, or other Posts that defend the Passage of the Ditch, or the like, they have a dreadful Effect

Cartridge-Box, is a Tin Case with Partitions, to carry the Cartridges above-mention'd in

Cascabel The very hindmost Knob of the Cannon, or utmost Part of the Breech

Castle, in French, *Chasteau* A Place strong, either by Art or Nature, whether in a City, or in the Country, to keep the People in Obedience. A sort of a little Citadel

Cavalier, or *Mount* A great Elevation or heap of Earth, sometimes round, and sometimes a long Square; on the Top whereof is a Platform, with a Parapet to cover the Cannon planted on it The height of it must be proportionable to that part of the Enemies Ground or Works it is designed to overlook or command Those which are rais'd upon the Enclosure of any Place, whether in the

middle

middle of the Curtin, or in the Gorge of a Bastion are generally 15 or 18 Foot higher than the *Terre-plein* of the Rampart The breadth of them is to be regulated by the number of Cannon design'd to be planted on them, observing that there must be ten or twelve Foot Distance allow'd between every two Guns for the Conveniency of the Gunners

Cavalry That Body of Soldiers that serves and fights on Horse-back These are either Regimented, or Independent Troops, as the Troops of Guards, and in *France* the *Gendarmes* and Musketeers a Horse-back All these upon Service are drawn up in Bodies, call'd Squadrons

Cavin A Hollow, fit to cover Troops, and facilitate their Approach to a Place. If it be within Musket-shot, it is a Place of Arms ready made to hand, and a Conveniency for opening the Trenches, out of fear of the Enemies Shot

Cazematte A Platform in that Part of the Flank of a Bastion next the Curtin, somewhat retir'd, or drawn back towards the Capital of the Bastion. Sometimes it consists of three Platforms, one above another, the *Terre-plain* of the Bastion being the highest for which Reason the *French* give the others the Name of *Places Basses*, or Low Places Behind their Parapet which fronts along the Line of the Flank, there are Guns planted, loaded with Cartridges of small Shot,to scour along the Ditch, and these Guns are co- ver'd from the Enemies Betteries by Earth-Works, fac'd or lin'd with Wall, and call'd *Orillons* or *Epaulments* The *Cazematte* is the most excellent Defence a Place can have

Cazernes Little Rooms, or Lodg- ments generally built between the Ram- part and Houses of a fortify'd Town, to quarter Soldiers for the Ease of the In- habitants. There are generally two Beds in each Cazern for six Soldiers to lie, three and three, but so that the third Part being always upon Guard, there are but four left in the Cavern, or two in a Bed

Center The middle Point of any Work or Body of Men The Pikes are in the Center of the Battalion, the youngest Regiments in the Center of the Army From the Center of a Place, are drawn the first Lines to lay down the Form of Fortification.

Chace of a Gun The whole length

Chain, is nothing but a sort of Wire- Chain divided into Links of an equal length, which Engineers make use of for setting out Works on the Ground, be- cause the Line is apt both to shrink and give way

Chain-shot Vide *Shot*

Chamade A signal made by the Enemy, either by beat of Drum, or sound of Trumpet, when they have any Matter

to

to propose; otherwise call'd, *To sound or beat a Parly*, which is the more proper English But *Chamade* begins to grow familiar, as do all other Terms in Martial Affairs The Besiegers beat the *Chamade* or *Parley*, to have Leave to bury their Dead The Besieged beat the *Chamade* or *Parley*, and *Capitulate*

Chamber of a Gun That Part where the Powder and Shot lies

Chamber of a Mine, Is the Place where the Powder is laid, at the End of the Gallery or Passage, and is never above six Foot square every way But if the Mine be to blow up a hollow or voided Bastion, and consequently the Thinness of it next the Place giving Occasion to fear lest the Besieg'd give the Mine vent that Way, then the Top of the Chamber is cut in a Cross, or like a *Bonnet a Prestre*, or Priest's Cap, that the Fire may take vent upwards The Powder is generally laid in Barrils, unless the Ground be very dry, and then it is in Bags

Chandeliers Wooden Frames, large and strong, to pile Faggots against, one upon another, to cover the Workmen instead of a Parapet These are to remove from Place to Place, as Occasion requires, upon sudden Emergencies, or whilst the Trenches are digging

Charge A Charge is the Quantity of Powder and Ball fit for any Piece, great or small.

To charge a Piece, Is to put in the proper Quantity of Powder and Ball

To charge to the Right or Left, Is for the Pikemen to lay their Pikes on their Left Arms level Breast high, holding the Butt Ends in their Right, to oppose the Horse or other Foot that shall attempt to break in upon them The Musketeers, at the Word of Command, hold their Muskets rested, the Cocks in their Right Hands and the Barrils resting on their Left

Chargers, Are either Bandaleers or Flasks that contain the Powder

Charg'd Cylinder, or *Chamber* The Part of a Cannon which contains the Powder and Shot

Chausse, Res de Chausse The Level of the Field, the plain Ground

Chausse Traps Vide *Crows-Feet*

Chemin Couvert Vide *Covert-way*

Chemin des Rondes, or Way of the Rounds. A Space between the Rampart and the low Parapet under it, for the Rounds to go about It is the same as the *Fausse Braye*. Vide *Fausse Braye*

Chemise A Word almost out of Date formerly signifying the Wall that faced or lined a Work of Earth, especially when the Soil was sandy and loose, and therefore could not support it self, without allowing it too great a *Talus* or Stoop

Chevaux de Frise, or *Horse de Frise* The same as Turnpikes, only some will have it, that the *Chevaux* are made stronger than

than the *Turnpikes*, but there is no other Difference but in the Language, one being the *French*, the other the *English* Name, yet both indifferently now us'd in *England*, and the *French* rather the most. Vide *Turnpike*

Cinquain An ancient Order of Battle, to draw up 5 Batalions, so that they may make three Lines, that is, a Van, Main Body, and Body of Reserve Supposing the Five Battalions to be in a Line, the 2d and 4th advance and form the Van, the 3d falls back for the Rear-Guard, or Body of Reserve, the 1st and 5th for the main Body upon the same Ground. Then every Batalion ought to have a Squadron of Horse on its Right, and another on its Left Any Number of Regiments produc'd by the Multiplication of the Number 5, as 10, 15, 20, *&c* may be drawn up in the same Manner

Circumvallation A Line, or Trench, with a Parapet, thrown up by the Besiegers, a Cannon-shot from the Place, encompassing all their Camp, to defend it against any Army that may attempt to relieve the Place, so that the Army besieging lies between the two Lines of Contravallation, and Circumvallation, the former against the Besieg'd and the latter against those that shall pretend to relieve them. The Line of Circumvallation is generally about seven Foot deep, and about twelve Foot broad The Parapet runs quite round the Top of it, and at certain Distances it is strengthen'd with Redoubts and small Forts The Line of Circumvallation must never run along the Foot of a rising Ground, because if an Enemy shall possess himself of the height, he might plant Cannon there, and command the Line

Citadel, Is a Fort with four, five, or six Bastions, rais'd on the most advantageous Ground about a City, the better to command it, and divided from it by an *Esplanade*, or open Space, the better to hinder the Approach of an Enemy So that the Citadel defends the Inhabitants if they continue in their Duty, and punishes them if they revolt. Besiegers always attack the City first, that being Masters of it, they may cover themselves the better against the Fire of the Citadel

Clates, are the same as commonly we call *Wattles*, being made of strong Stakes, interwoven with Oziers, or other small pliable Twigs, and the closer the better They are generally about 5 or 6 Foot long, and 3 or 3 and a half broad The Use of them is to cover Lodgments overhead with much Earth heap'd on them, to secure the Men against the Fire works, and Stones thrown by the Besieg'd They are also cast into a Ditch that has been drein'd, for the Besiegers to pass over on them without sticking in the Mud

To clear the Trenches To beat out those that are to guard them with a vigorous Sally from the Place besieg'd, to throw

down

own the Parapet, fill the Trench, and
l the Cannon

To Cloy Guns Vide *To Nail*

Cock The Cock of any Fire-Arm is
at which holds the Flint, and being
wn back, stands till the Trigger mo-
ng the Spring falls with such force
beats open the Pan, and the Flint
ecting with the Steel over the Pan,
ikes Fire, which takes the Powder in
e Pan, and so through the Touch-hole
discharges the Piece

To Cock a Musket or Pistol; Is to bend
e Cock backwards, in order to fire the
ece by drawing back the Trigger

The Cock half bent, Is the usual standing
it, when neither cock'd nor quite
wn

Coffre A Depth sunk in the bottom of
ry Ditch, of the whole breadth of the
d Ditch from side to side, and cover'd
th Joists, rais'd two Foot above the
tom of the Ditch, which rising serves
tead of a Parapet, with Loop-holes in
and this Work being made at leisure
the Besieg'd, it serves to fire on the
iegers when they attempt to cross
Ditch The Breadth of the *Coffre* is
ut 15 or 18 Foot, and the depth six
even Only its Length distinguishes
om the *Caponniere*, which does not
h the whole breadth of the Ditch,
it differs from the *Traverse* and *Gale-*
in that these two are made by the Be-
ers, and the *Coffre* by the Besieg'd

The

The Besiegers *Epaul*, or cover themselv against the *Coffers*, throwing up the Ea on that Side, on which the Musketee in it fire

Coffre, Is also taken for the same *Caisson* Vide *Caisson*

Colonel The Commander in Chief o Regiment either of Horse, Foot, Dragoons in *England*, but in *France* *Spain*, they call the Colonels of Hor *Master de Camp* Colonels of Foot Place, and command one another accor ing to the Antiquity of their Regimen and not of their Commissions, but th of Horse on the contrary, according the Dates of their Commissions, with regard to the Antiquity of the Re ments Their Post at the Head of Regiments is three Paces before the C tains Sometimes there are Colone General of Horse, Foot, and Dragoo whose Authority extends over each these Bodies

Column The long File or Row Troops, or of Baggage, of an Army its march So to march in a Column to march a great depth, or in a long Fi instead of making a large Front An A my marches in one, two, three, or mo Columns, according as the Ground w allow, and the General sees expedient.

Command, *Word of Command* T Terms us'd by Officers in Exercise upon Service,

Command

Commanding Ground A Rising Ground, which overlooks any Post, or strong Place There are three sorts of Commanding Grounds

A Front Commanding Ground A height opposite to the Face of the Post which plays upon its Front

A Reverse Commanding-Ground An Eminence which plays upon the back of a Post

An Enfilade Commanding-Ground, or *Curtain Commanding-Ground* A high Place which with its Shot scours all the length of a straight Line

Commissary-General of the Musters, or *Muster Master General* Takes Account of the Strength of every Regiment, reviews them, sees the Horse be well mounted, and all Men well arm'd and accoutred

Commissary-General of Provisions, Has the Charge of furnishing the Army with all sorts of Provisions, and must be very vigilant and industrious, that they may never suffer Want

Commission The Authority by which every Officer acts in his Post, sign'd by the King, or by his General, if he be impower'd

Commission-Officers Vide *Officers*

Company A small Body of Foot, the Number never fix'd, commanded by a Captain Generally two Thirds of the Company are arm'd with Muskets, and the rest with Pikes, but this Particular may also vary

Independent

Independent Company That which is not incorporated in a Regiment

Complement of the Curtin, Is that part of the interior Side which forms the Demi-Gorge

Contravallation A Trench with a Parapet the Besiegers cover themselves with next the Place besieg'd, to defend them against the Sallies of the Garison, so that the Army forming a Siege, lies between the Lines of Circumvallation and Contravallation This Line is carry'd on without Musket-Shot of the Town, and sometimes goes quite round it, sometimes not, according as the General sees occasion

Contre-Queue d'yronde, or *Counter-Swallows-Tail* An Outwork in the form of a single *Tenaille*, wider next the Place, that is, at the Gorge, than at the Head, or next the Campaign Which is the contrary in the *Queue d'yronde*, or *Swallows-Tail*, this being widest at the Head The Sides of the *Contre-Queue* are not so well flank'd from the Place as those of the *Queue d'yronde*, or *Swallows-Tail*, and therefore is not so good

Contribution An Imposition or Tax paid by all Frontier Countries, to redeem themselves from being plunder'd and destroy'd by the Enemy

Conversion, as *Wheel by Conversion* is the same among the Horse, as Wheeling among the Foot, that is, the whole Front turning to the Right or Left still keeping

th

eir Order, making a fourth Part of Circle in their Motion, for in wheeling to the Right, the right-hand Man nds upon the same Ground only fang to the Right, whilst all the rest move ward more or less as they are near or from him, to come up and make an ual Front to the Right

Convoy A Supply of Men, Money, mmunitions and Provisions, convey'd to a Town, or to an Army, or the Bo- of Men that marches to secure any ng from the Enemy.

Copper Boats Vide *Bridge*.

Corbeilles. Vide *Baskets*

Cordean A Line divided into Fathoms, et, &c to mark Out-works on the ound us'd by Engineers.

Cordon; Is a putting out of Stone comnly round, running round the Wall wards the Top

Coridor Vide *Covert-way*

Cornet A Commission-Officer belong- to every Troop of Horse, subordi- e to the Captain and Lieutenant, uivalent to the Ensign among the ot

Cornish-Ring of a Gun The next Ring m the Muzzle backwards

Corns of Powder; Are the small Grains Gunpowder consists of

Corporal An Inferior Officer of Foot, o has charge of one of the Divisions a Company, places and relieves Sen- els, and keeps good order in the *Corps*

de

de Garde. He receives the Word of th Inferior Rounds, that pass by his Co *de Garde* Every Company, if sm has three Corporals, but more if n merous

Corps de Garde A Post, someti under Covert, and sometimes in t open Air, to receive a Number of M who are reliev'd from time to ti to watch in their Turns for the Sec rity of some more considerable Po This Word *Corps de Garde* does n only signify the Post, but the M in it

Corps de Bataille. The main Bo of an Army drawn up for Ba whereof the first Line is call'd the *V* the second the *Corps de Bataille*, *Main Battle*, and the third the *Corps de* *serve, Body of Reserve*, or *Rear-Guard* V *Battle*

Corps de Reserve Vide *Line of Ba* and *Rear-Guard*

Covert-way In French, *Chemin Cou* or *Corridor* A Space of Ground le with the Field upon the Edge of Ditch, three or four Fathom wide, cover'd with a Parapet or Brest w running all round the Moat, and slop gently towards the Campaign It also a Foot-bank One of the grea Difficulties in a Siege, is to make a Lo ment on the *Covert-way*, because ge rally the Besieged pallisade it along Middle, and undermine it on all Si

T

This is commonly call'd the *Counter-scarp*, because it is on the Edge of it

Counter-Approaches Lines or Trenches carried on by the Besieged, when they come out to attack the Lines of the Besiegers in form

Counter Battery A Battery that plays upon another

Counter-Guard In French, *Contre-garde*, or *Envelope* A small Rampart with a Parapet and Ditch to cover some part of the Body of the Place There are Counter-Guards of several Shapes, and differently situated Those rais'd before the Point of a Bastion, consist of Two Faces, making an Angle Saillant, and parallel to the Faces of the Bastion Those which cover one of the Faces of the Bastion, are shap'd like a Demi-Bastion, with a Parapet upon the Face and Capital, but none on the Flank, which must be open, and expos'd to the Fire of the Place This Name of *Counter-Guard*, is not much in use at present among Engineers, who call it an *Envelope* Count *Pagan* calls that Work about any Place beyond the Great Ditch, the *Counter-Guard*, or Great *Counterscarp* But there is no Place fortified according to his Method, because of the excessive Charge it requires. Vide *Envelope*

Counter-Line Vide *Contravallation*.

Countermarch When the Files countermarch, it changes the Face or Front of the Battalion, and when Ranks counter-march,

march, it is exchanging the Wings of the Battalion The Files countermarch to bring those that are in the Front to the Rear, which is proper when a Battalion is charg'd in the Rear, and the Commander would have the File-Leaders who are generally chosen Men, take the Place of the Bringers up The Ranks countermarch, when it is requir'd that one Wing of the Battalion should exchange its Ground with the other

Countermine A Well, or Hole, sunk into the Ground, from which a Gallery or Branch runs out under Ground, to seek out the Enemies Mine, and disappoint it

Counterscarp, is properly the *Talus*, or Slope of the Ditch, on the farther side from the Place, and facing it. But by this Name is commonly meant the *Covert-way* and *Glacis*, and in this Sense it is said the Enemy attack'd the Counterscarp or lodg'd themselves on the Counterscarp

Counterscarp, *Ditch of the Counterscarp* Vide *Avant Fosse*

Counter-Trenches; Are Trenches cast up against the Besiegers, and consequently have their Parapet towards them, and are enfiladed from several parts of the Place, to hinder the Enemy from making use of them when they are Masters of them But Care must be taken that they be not enfiladed, nor commanded by any Eminence possess'd by the Enemy

Croat

Croat, properly the People of *Croatia*. But in *France* there is a Regiment o call'd, because at first they were of hat Nation, tho' now they are all *French*, s are those they still call the *Scotch Gendarmes* These *Croats* are commanded upn all desperate Service, and therefore n a Battle they are posted on the Wings, little advanc'd before the other Squarons, upon the Line with the Draoons

Crown-Work, in French, *Ouvrage a ouronn*. An Out-work that takes up ore Ground than any other It is ade up of a large Gorge, and two Sides erminating towards the Campaign in o Demi-Bastions, each of which is oyn'd by a particular Curtin to a whole astion that is at the Head of the Work rown-Works are made to cover some rge Spot of Ground, to secure some sing Ground, or to defend the Head of Camp that is intrench'd

Crows-Feet, Caultrops, or *Chaussetrapes* our-pointed Irons so made, that what ay soever they fall, one Point is up, ing 2, 3, or 4 Inches long; the short es to strew on Bridges or Planks, the nger on the Earth Both to incomode the Cavalry, that they may not pproach without great Difficulty, the oint that sticks up running into the orses Feet

A Cube, is a solid Body, every way uare.

Cubical.

Cubical The Body that is so sol[id] and square as a cubical Foot, that is Foot square every way of any Sub[-] stance

Cuirassiers Horse that wear Armou[r]

Culverin, of the least Size A Gu[n] 5 Inches Diameter in the Bore, 4 Pounds weight, takes a Charge of Pounds of Powder, and carries a Ball Inches and 6 Eights Diameter and Pounds Weight, and Random shot Paces

Culverin Ordinary, Is 5 Inches 2 Eigh[ts] Diameter in the Bore, 4500 Poun[ds] Weight, takes 11 Pounds 6 Ounces Charg[e] of Powder, and carries a Ball 5 Inches Di[-] ameter, and 17 Pounds 5 Ounces Weigh[t]

Culverin, of the largest Size, Is 5 Inch[es] 4 Eights Diameter in the Bore, 480[0] Pounds Weight, takes a Charge of Pounds 8 Ounces of Powder, and ca[r-] ries a Shot 5 Inches and 2 Eights Diam[e-] ter, and 20 Pounds Weight

Curtin That Part of the Wall, Rampart, that lies between two Bastio[ns] Besiegers seldom carry on their Atta[cks] against it, because it is the best flank[ed] of any Part

Cuttings off Vide *Retrenchments.*

Cuvette A deeper Trench cut alo[ng] the middle of the dry Ditch, and gen[e-] rally carry'd down till there be Wa[ter] to fill it This is a Ditch within t[he] Ditch, and runs all the Length of it, t[he] better to keep off the Enemy T[he]

Bread[th]

adth of it ought to be 18 or 20
t

ylinder Concave Cylinder of a Gun, he hollow length of a Piece

harged Cylinder The Chamber, or that which receives the Charge of Powder Shot

acant Cylinder That part of the Hol- which remains empty when the Gun harg'd

D.

DEcagon A Figure that has ten Sides, and as many Angles, capable of ng fortify'd with ten Bastions

o d camp To raise the Camp, to ak up from the Place where the Army encamp'd, and march away

Defence *Line of Defence* Vide *Line*.

Defence of a Place All those Parts of a tification that flank other Parts, as *Parapets*, *Cazematttes*, or *Fausse-Brays*, ich face and defend those Posts that opposite to them It is almost impoi- e to fix the Miner to the Face of a tion, till the Defences of the opposite tion are ruin'd; that is, till the Para- of its Flank is beaten down, and Cannon in all Parts that can fire up- that Face which is attack'd are dis- unted

To be in a Posture of Defence, is to be dy and provided to oppose an Ene- my my As, Our Redoubt is in a good Posture of Defence; that is, the Work of it is finish'd, and it can oppose an Enemy

Defile. A narrow Pass, or Way, where Troops cannot march but by making a small Front; and therefore are forc'd to file off, which gives the Enemy an Opportunity of charging them more advantageously, because the Rear cannot come up to relieve the Front

Degree Tho' this Term properly belongs to Geometry, it is so often us'd in Fortification, that it will not be improper to declare it as a small Part of the Arch of a Circle, whereof every Circle contains 360, which serve to measure the Content of the Angle So we say, the Angle is of 20, of 50, or of 70 Degrees or more Vide *Angle.*

Demi Bastion Vide *Bastion*

Demi-Cannon Lowest A Great Gun that carries a Ball of 30 Pounds weight, and 6 Inches Diameter. Its Charge of Powder 14 Pounds. It shoots point-blank 156 Paces The Weight of it [...] Pounds, the Length 11 Foot, the Diameter of the Bore 6 Inches 2 Eighth Parts.

Demi-Cannon Ordinary A great Gun [...] Inches four Eights Diameter in the Bore, 12 Foot long, weight 5600 lb. takes a Charge of 17 Pounds 8 Ounces of Powder, carries a Shot six Inches one Sixth

Diameter and 32 Pounds Weight, and hoots point-blank 162 Paces

Dem-Cannon of the greatest Size A Gun 6 Inches, and 6 Eight Parts Diameter in the Bore, 12 Foot long, 6000 Pounds Weight; akes a Charge of 18 Pounds of Powder; arries a Ball 6 Inches 5 Eights Diameter, and 36 Pounds Weight The Piece hoots point-blank 180 Paces

Demi-Culverin, of the lowest Size A Gun Inches 2 Eights Diameter in the Bore, o Foot long, 2000 Pounds Weight, kes a Charge of 6 Pounds 4 Ounces of owder, carries a Ball 4 Inches Diameter, and 9 Pounds Weight, and shoots oint-blank 174 Paces

Demi-Culverin Ordinary A Gun 4 Inches Eights Diameter in the Bore, 10 Foot ong, 2700 Pounds Weight, charg'd with Pounds 4 Ounces of Powder, carries Ball 4 Inches two Eights Diameter, nd 10 Pounds 11 Ounces Weight It oots point-blank 175 Paces

Demi-Culverin, elder Sort A Gun 4 Inches d 6 Eights Diameter in the Bore, ten oot one Third in length, 3000 Pounds Weight, charg'd with eight Pounds eight unces of Powder and carries a Ball 4 ches 4 Eight Parts Diameter, and 12 unds 11 Ounces Weight Its point-ank shot 178 Paces

Demi-Gorge Half the Gorge, or Enance into the Bastion, not taken direct-from Angle to Angle where the Baon joyns to the Curtin but from the

Angle of the Flank to the Center of the Bastion, or Angle the two Curtins would make, were they protracted to meet in the Bastion Vide *Gorge*, as *D I.* and *D* [illegible] *Fig* 1

Depth of a Squadron or Batalion The number of Men there is in the File. That of a Squadron is always three, and that of a Batalion generally six So we say, the Batalion is drawn up six deep, or five deep

Descents into the Ditch Trenches or Cuts made by way of *Sappe*, in the Ground of the Counterscarp, under the *Covert-way*, and cover'd with Madriers, that is, Planks, or with Clays, that is large Wattles close bound together, and well loaded with Earth to secure them against Fire In Ditches that are full of Water, the Descent is made even to the Superficies of the Water, and then the Ditch is fill'd with Faggots fast bound and cover'd with Earth In dry Ditches the *Sappe* is carry'd down to the bottom, and they make *Traverses* in it, either to lodge themselves, or secure the Miner

Deserter A Soldier that runs away to the Enemy, or that quits the Service without Leave, or runs from one Regiment to another Deserters are punish'd with Death.

Detachment A number of Men drawn out of one or more greater Bodies, either to mount Guards, make an Attack, or other Service Sometim

Flying Army is made up of Detachments

To Dismount The vulgar and general Meaning is, to unhorse ; as, to dismount Cavalry : But,

To Dismount Cannon, Is to throw it off the Carriages, or break and render them unfit for Service

Dispart To dispart a Cannon, is to set a Mark on the Muzzle-Ring to be of an equal height or level with the Base-Ring, so that a Line drawn between them shall be parallel to the Axis of the Concave Cylinder, for the Gunner to take Aim by it at the Mark he is to shoot; for the Bore and this being parallel, the Aim taken by it must be true.

Ditch, Vide *Moat*

Ditch of the Counterscarp. Vide *Avant-fosse*

Divisions, Are the several Parcels into which a Batalion is divided in marching, consisting generally of about 6 Files each, and led by the Lieutenants and Ensigns, the Captains marching in the Front and Rear The Divisions of an Army are the Brigades

Dodecagon A Figure that has twelve Sides, and as many Angles, capable of being fortifi'd with the same number of Bastions.

Double Tenaille. Vide *Tenaille*.

To Double To put two Ranks into one, or two Files into one, according as the Word of Command expresses it As, Double

ble your Ranks, is for the second, four and sixth Ranks to march into the fi third, and fifth, so that of six Ranks t make but three, leaving double the Int val there was between them before, wh is not so when they double by half Fi because then three Ranks stand togeth and the three others come up to dou them; that is, the first, second, third are doubled by the fourth, fifth sixth, or the contrary Double y Files, is for every other File to ma into that which is next to it on the Ri or Left, as the Word of Command rects, and then the six Ranks are tu into twelve, the Men standing tw deep, and the Distance between the F is double what it was before

Dragoons. Musketeers mounted, serve sometimes a Foot, and sometim Horse-back, being always ready upon thing that requires Expedition, as b able to keep pace with the Horse, and the Service of Foot In Battle, or u Attacks, they are commonly the *En Perdus*, or Forlorn, being the first fall on. In the Field, they encamp e at the Head of the Army, or on Wings, to cover the others, and be first at their Arms They have Con like the Horse, and Sergeants like Foot, but are look'd upon as Foot T Martial Musick, Drums and Haut-b

Draw-Bridge Vide *Bridge*

D

Drein A Trench cut to draw the
ter out of a Moat As soon as the
at is drein'd, they cast into it Clays
er'd with Earth, or Bundles of Rushes
h Planks on them, to make them a
age over the Mud

Droit Attacks Vide *Attacks*

Drum Either the Martial Instrumen
f us'd by Foot and Dragoons, or the
n that beats it, which is done after se-
al Manners, either to give Notice to
Troops of what they are to do, or to
and Liberty to make some Proposal to
Enemy Every Regiment of Foot
a Drum-Major, who commands all
rest, and every Company has one or
. To beat the General, to give No-
to the Forces that they are to march.
beat the Troop, to order the Men to
ir to their Colours To beat a March,
command them to move To beat
Tat-to, to order all to retire to their
rters To beat the *Reveille*, at break
ay to give Leave to come out of Quar-
To beat a Charge, a Signal to fall
n the Enemy To beat a Retreat, to
off from the Enemy To beat to
s, for Soldiers that are dispers'd to
ir to them To beat an Alarm, to
Notice of some sudden Danger that
nay be in a Readiness To beat a
y, or Chamade a Signal to demand
Conference with the Enemy When
alion is drawn up, the Drums are
e Flanks and when it marches by

Divisions or Sub-Divisions, they ma[y] between them.

Duty. The Exercise of those Functio[ns] that belong to a Soldier, yet with [a] nice Distinction, That Duty is coun[ted] Mounting Guards, and the like, wh[en] there is not an Enemy directly to be [en]gag'd, for when they march to meet [the] Enemy, it is call'd *going upon Service*

E

E*Arth Bags.* Vide *Canvas Bags*

Echarpe. Battery en Echarpe V[ide] *Battery*

Echaugette Vide *Gueritte.*

Elder Batalion, or *Officer*. The Batal[ion] is counted elder than another by the T[ime] since it was rais'd, and according to [its] standing has the Post of Honour, [and] Officers are accounted elder than oth[ers] not by their Age, or the Time they [have] been Soldiers, but by the Date of t[heir] Commission, and accordingly they ar[e to] take their Posts *See* more of this u[nder] the Word *Seniority*

Embrazures The Gaps or Loop-ho[les] left open in a Parapet for the Cannon [to] fire through. The usual Distance betw[een] the Embrazures is generally 12 Foot, [for] the Conveniency of the Gunners, [and] that the Parapet may not be too m[uch] weaken'd. Every Embrazure is three F[oot] above the Platform next to the Can[non,] and a Foot and half next the Camp[aign] to sink the Muzzle, and play low. Each of them is about 3 Foot wide within, and about 6 or 7 without, for the Conveniency of traversing the Guns.

Eminence, or *Height* A Rising Ground that over-looks and commands that under it.

Empattement The same as *Talus* Vide *Talus*.

Enfans perdus Men detach'd from several Regiments, or otherwise appointed to give the first on-set in Battle, or at an Attack upon a Place besieg d, so call'd because of the eminent Danger they are expos'd to In English, they are commonly call'd, *The Forlorn.*

Enfilade The Situation of a Post, which can discover and scour all the Length of a Streight Line, which by that means is rendred almost defenceless

To Enfile, or *Enfilade* the Curtin or Rampart To sweep the whole Length of it with the Shot

Engineer A Person well skill d in the Art of contriving all sorts of Forts, and other Works, judicious in finding out Faults in all Fortifications, and mending them, and knowing how to attack and defend all sorts of Posts

Enneagon A Figure that has nine Sides and as many Angles, capable of being fortify'd with the same number of Bastions

Ensign The Officer that carries the Colours among the Foot, and is the last Commission-Officer in the Company, being subordinate to the Captain and Lieutenant The Ensign's Post is at the Head of the Pikes He is to dye rather th[an] lose his Colours

Envelope A Work of Earth rais'd sometimes in the Ditch of a Place, sometimes beyond the Ditch, sometimes like a plain Parapet, and sometimes like a little Rampart with a Parapet to it *Envelopes* are generally made when weak Places are cover'd only with bare Lines, and either they cannot, or will not stretch out towards the Campaign with Half-moons, Horn-works or the like Works which require much Ground The *Envelopes* in a Ditch, [are] sometimes call'd *Sillons*, *Counter-Gardes*, *Conserves* or *Lunettes* See all these Words

Epaule, or Shoulder of a Bastion The space contain'd by the Angle, made by the Union of the Face and Flank, whence that Angle is call'd, *The Angle of the Epaule*

Epaulment A Work to a Side, or sideways, made either of Earth thrown up of Bags of Earth, of Gabions, or of Fascines and Earth The [Epau]*lments* of the Places of Arms for the Cavalry behind the Trenches, are generally only of Fascines and Earth

Epaulment, is also taken for a *Demi-Bastion* Vide *Bastion*

Epaulment, or Square *Orillon* A Mass of Earth almost Square, and fac'd or lin'd with a Wall to cover the Cannon of [a] *Cazematte* Vide *Orillon*

Equilateral A Figure that has all its Sides equal

Escalade. Vide *Scalade*

Escarp. Vide *Scarp*

Escouade, generally is the Third Part of a Company of Foot, so divided for mounting of Guards, and relieving one another, Equivalent to a Brigade of Horse

Esplanade It properly signifies the Glacis of the Counterscarp, but begins to be antiquated in that Sense, and is now only taken for the empty Space between the Glacis of a Citadel, and the first Houses of a Town

Etoile Vide *Star Redoubt*

Etappe An allowance of Provisions, and Forage, for Soldiers in their March through the Kingdom to or from Winter-quarters

Etappier One that contracts with a Country, or Territory, for furnishing Troops in their March with Provisions and Forage They are to deliver the *Etappe* to the Majors of Horse or Foot, and in their Absence to the Quatermasters of each Troop of Horse, or Sergeants of the Company of Foot *Etappiers* are forbid giving Soldiers their *Etappe* in Money Somtimes the *Etappiers* and Officers compound for a Sum of Money, and oblige the Men to make two Days March in one, which is great harassing of Men and Horses, and a notorious Fraud

Evolutions. The Motions made by a Body of Men in changing their Posture, or Form of Drawing up, to make good the Ground they are on, or possess them-

 selves

selves of another, that they may either attack the Enemy, or receive his onset more advantageously The *Evolutions* are doubling of Ranks or Files, Counter marches and Wheelings

Exercise The Practice of all those Motions, and Actions, and Management of Arms, a Soldier is to be perfect in, to be fit for Service, and make him understand how to Attack and Defend.

F

FAce of a Bastion The two foremost Sides reaching from the Flanks to the Point of the Bastion where they meet, are call'd the *Faces* These are commonly the first undermin'd, because they reach farthest out, and are least flank'd, and therefore weakest.

Face of a Place, call'd also the *Tenaille* of the Place. The Interval between the Points of two Neighbouring Bastions, containing the Curtin, the two Flanks, and the two Faces of the Bastions that look upon one another.

Face prolong'd, or *extended* Is that part of the Line of Defence Razant, which is terminated by the Curtin, and the Angle of the *Epaul*; that is, it is the Line of Defence Razant, diminish'd by the Face of the Bastion

Facings To Face, is to look towards such a Side, or to turn to it; as Face to the

the Right, or to the Left, is to turn the Face and whole Body that way

Faggots The *French* call them *Passevolans* Are Men hir'd to Muster, by Officers whose Companies are not full, to cheat the King of so many Men's Pay The King of *France* has ordered, That any who shall be found so to pass in Musters, if discover'd, have a *Flower-de-luce* burnt upon their Cheek, and lose their Arms and Equipage

Faggots are also the same as *Fascines*.

Falcon Vide *Faucon*

Falconet Vide *Fauconet*

False Alarm Vide *Alarm*

False Attack. Vide *Attack*

Fanion A Banner carry'd by a Servant belonging to each Brigade of Horse and, Foot, at the Head of the Baggage of each Brigade, to keep good order, and prevent Confusion in the March It is made of Stuff, of the Colour of the Brigadiers, or the Commanding Officer's Livery. It is a Corruption of *Gonfanon*, which in *Italian* signifies a Banner

Fascines, Are Faggots of small Wood, which distinguishes them from the *Saucissons*, made of bigger Branches of Trees. *Fascines* are greater or less, according to the several Uses they are put to Those that are to be pitch'd, to burn a Lodgment, Gallery, or other Work of the Enemy's, are but a Foot and a half long; but those that are for making *Epaulments* or

Chan-

Chandeliers, or to raise Works, or fill up wet Ditches, must be between two and three Foot in thickness, and four Foot long, and being to be loaded with much Earth to make them more solid, and prevent their being fir'd, they are bound at both Ends as well as in the Middle. The Enemy has no way to destroy them, but by fire, to prevent which, they are either loaded with Earth, as has been said, or cover'd with raw Hides.

A Faucon, or *Falcon*. A small Cannon, 2 Inches and 6 Eights Diameter in the Bore, 7 Foot long, weighing 750 Pounds, takes a Charge of 2 Pounds 4 Ounces of Powder, and carries a Ball 2 Inches and 5 Eights Diameter, and 2 Pounds 8 Ounces Weight. It's point-blank Shot 130 Paces.

A Fauconet, or *Falconet*. A very small Piece of Cannon, 2 Inches and 2 Eights Diameter in the Bore, 6 Foot long, weighing 400 Weight, takes a Charge of one Pound 4 Ounces of Powder, and carries a Bullet 2 Inches and 1 Eight Diameter and 1 Pound 5 Ounces Weight. Its point-blank Shot 90 Paces.

Fausse-Braye, Chemin des Rondes, Basse Enceinte, or *Lower Enclosure*, Is a space about the breadth of 2 or 3 Fathoms, round the Foot of the Rampart, on the out-side, defended by a Parapet, which parts it from the *Berme*, or *Foreland*, and the Edge of the Ditch. The Design of the *Fausse-Braye*, is to defend the *Moat*, but they are useless where

where Ramparts are fac'd or lin'd with Wall, because of the Rubbish the Cannon beats down into them. Therefore most Engineers will have none before the Faces of the Bastions, where the Breach is commonly made, because the Ruins falling, the *Fausse Braye* make the ascent to the Breach the easier, and what flies from the Faces, kills the Soldiers that are to defend them.

Fichant. Vide *Line of Defence Fichant.*

Field Officer. Vide *Officer.*

File. The strait Line Soldiers make that stand one before another, which is the depth of the Batallion or Squadron, and thus distinguish'd from the Rank, where the Men stand Side by Side, and make the length of the Batalion or Squadron. Among the Foot, the Files are six deep, among the Horse, but three. The Files must be strait, and parallel to one another. To double Files, is to put two Files into one, which makes the depth of the Batalion double what it was, not in space of Ground, but in number of Men, and also doubles the Intervals between the Files, making the Ranks look thin. The Men in a File are distinguish'd by the several Names of File-leaders, Half-files, and Bringers up. If a Batalion be drawn up Eight deep, there may be Quarter-files, but this is not usual.

File-Leaders. The Men that compose the Front, or first Rank of a Batalion, being the first of every File.

To File off To fall off from marching in a spacious Front, and march in length by Files When a Regiment is marching in full Front, and comes to a narrow Pass, it may march off by Divisions, or Subdivisions, or file off from the Right or Left, or as the Ground requires

Fire To Fire To discharge Fire-Arms

Fire-Arms Under this Name are comprehended all sorts of Arms that are charg'd with Powder and Ball, as Cannon, Muskets, Carabines, Pistols, Blunderbusses, *&c*

Running-Fire When Men drawn up for that purpose fire one after another, so that it runs the whole length of the Line or round a Town, or the like, which is us'd upon publick Occasions of Rejoycing

Fire-Ball Is made of ground Powder, Salt-petre, Brimstone, Camphire and Borace, all sprinkled with Oil, and moulded into a Mass, with Mutton Suet, ordinary Pitch and Greek Pitch, and made as big as an ordinary Granado. This is wrapp'd up in Tow, with a Sheet of strong Paper over it To fire it, they make a Hole into it with a Bodkin, into which they put some Priming that will burn slow This they cast into any Works they would discover in the Night time

Fire-Lock; Is a Piece that is fir'd with the Flint that is fast'ned to the Cock, whereas formerly Match-locks were most in use, fixing a Match to the Cock

Fire-Master A Person that makes the ...zes for Bombs, and Granadoes and ...er Fire-works

Flank That part of the Bastion which ...ches from the Curtin to the Face, and ...ends the opposite Face, the Flank, and ... Curtin

Oblique, or, *Second Flank* That part ... the Curtin that can see to scour the ...e of the opposite Bastion, and is the ...ance between the Lines *Razant*, and ...*ant*

Low, or *cover'd Flank*, or *Flank retire* ...e Platform of the *Cazematte*, which ... hid in the Bastion

Flank prolong'd, or *extended*; Is the stretch-... out of the Flank from the Angle of ... Epaule to the exterior Side, when ... Angle of the Flank is a right An-...

Flanks of a Batalion, or *Army* The ...s of them

To Flank To discover and fire upon ... Side. Any Fortification which has ... Defence but right forwards, is faulty, ... to make it compleat, one Part ought ... flank the other The Curtin is al-...ys the strongest part of any fortify'd ...ce, because it is flank'd by the two ...nks at the Ends of it.

Flank'd Angle The Angle form'd by ... two Faces of the Bastion, the Point ... the Bastion

Flask A Thing generally made of ...n to carry Powder in, with the Mea-

Measure of the Charge of the Piece to the Top of it

Flying-Army, or *Flying-Camp* Vide Camp

Flying Bridge Vide *Bridge*

Foot So absolutely taken, signifies those Bodies of Men that serve a-foot

Foot Is a measure divided into twelve Inches, being the 6th part of a Fathom the 5th of a Geometrical Pace, and us in Fortification

To be on the same foot with another is to be under the same Circumstances in point of Service

To gain or lose Ground foot by foot is to do it regularly and resolutely, defending every Thing to the utmost, or forcing it by dint of Art and Labour

Footbank, *Footstep* or *Banquette* A Step rais'd with Earth under the Parapet, to ... the Men to fire over it, about a Foot and half high, and three Foot wide The ... usually make two or three of them under the Parapets of little Forts and Redoubts

Foreland, *Barm*, *Berm* or *Lizier*, *Relais* *Retraite*, and *Pas de Souris* A small space of Ground between the Wall of a Place and the Moat, which the best Fortifications have not, because it is advantageous for the Enemy to come over the Moat and get footing, and therefore this is only left, where there is not enough to defray the Expence of Stone to face the foot of the Wall, in place whereof this helps to support it, and is generally from 3 to 8 or 10 Foot wide So says Sir ...

Moor, but the French say, this Space left to receive what the Enemy batters down from the Parapet, that it may not fill the Ditch For the more Security, this *Foreland* is generally pallisaded

The Forlorn Vide *Enfans perdus*

Forrage Hay, Straw, and Oats, for the Subsistence of Horses A Ration of Forrage, is the Day's Allowance for a Horse, which is 20 Pounds of Hay, 10 Pounds of Straw, and for want of Straw, Pounds of Hay

Fort A Work intrench'd on all Sides, design'd to secure some high Ground, or the Pass of a River, to make good any Spot of Ground, to fortify the Lines of Siege, and for many other Uses There are Forts of several Shapes and Sizes, according as the Ground requires Some are Whole-Bastions, others Demi-Bastions Some are Square, others Pentagons, *&c*

Fortification The Art of fortifying a Place, so that every Part may discover the Enemy in Front and Flank, and oppose the Depth of the Ditch, and the Height and Thickness of the Rampart against him, that so a small Body of Men within that Enclosure may advantageously oppose a great Army This same Word is also us'd, to signify all the Works that cover or defend a strong Place

Regular Fortification, is that which is made upon a Regular Polygon, whose sides do not exceed a Musket-shot, and which

which has all its Angles and Lines equ to one another, that is, has an equal For on all Sides

Irregular Fortification, is that which made on an irregular Polygon, which not equal Sides nor Angles, that is, not equal Force on all Sides. It is that which is made on a Regular P gon, when each Side of it is abov Musket-shot in length

Offensive Fortification Teaches a Ge ral how to take all Advantages for Troops, the manner of incamping, of besieging and taking of Troops

Defensive Fortification Shews a Go nour how to make the best of the Ga son committed to his Care, and to p vide all Things necessary for its Defe

Natural Fortification, consists in the tural Difficulty of Access to any P caus'd by Waters, Morasses, craggy steep Ascents, or the like, and teaches Engineer how to make the most of th

Artificial Fortification, is what an E neer thinks fit to add in Works, as R parts, Trenches, Bastions, Ravelins, H Moons, *&c* to supply the Defects of ture, and secure a Place against an Ene

Ancient Fortification, consists only in ces surrounded with Walls and To on them at Distances

Modern Fortification, is improv'd bey the Ancient, with the Addition of those several Works mention'd throu out this Dictionary

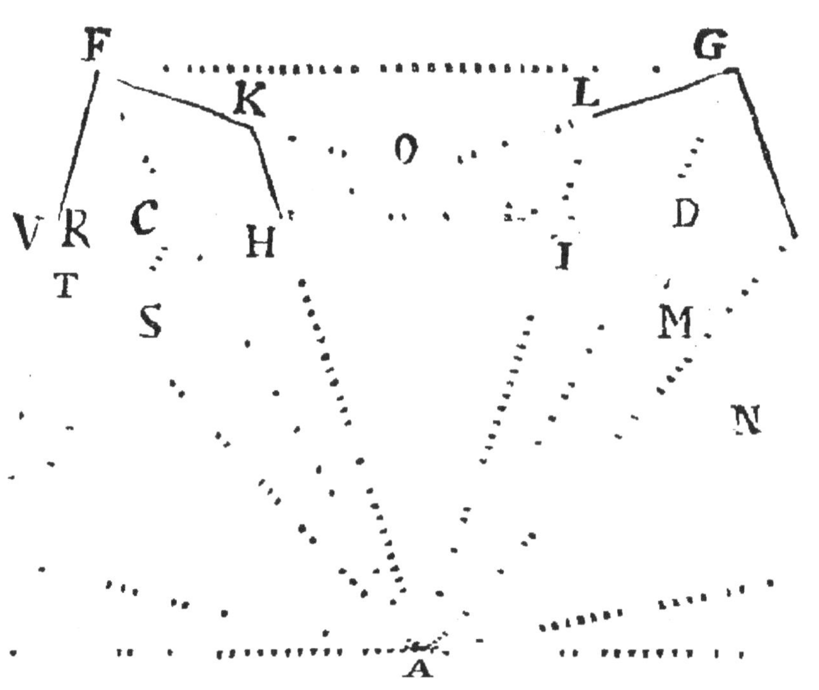

F
G
K
L
O
V
R
C
H
D
I
T
S
M
N
A

To Fortify Inwards, is to represent the Bastions within the Polygon propos'd to be fortify'd, and then that Polygon is call'd the *Exterior Polygon*, and each of its Sides the *Exterior Side*, terminating at the Points of the two nearest Bastions, as *F G* in *Fig* 1

To Fortify Outwards, is to represent the Bastion without the Polygon propos'd to be fortify'd, and then that Polygon is call'd the *Interior Polygon*, and each of its Sides the *Interior Side*, terminating in the Centers of the two nearest Bastions, as *C D* in *Fig* 1

Fortin A small Fort made like a Star, of 5 or more Points, to strengthen a Line of Circumvallation, or the like

Fosse Vide *Moat*

Foucade, *Fougade*, or *Fougasse* A *Fourneau*, or Chamber of a Mine made like a Well, eight or ten Foot wide, and ten or twelve in Depth, charg'd with Barrels or Bags of Powder, and prepar'd under a Post that is like to be lost It is cover'd with Earth, and fire put to it by a Train convey'd in a Pipe to another Post We could not keep our Footing on the Half-Moon we had gain'd, because the Enemy play'd two *Fougades*, which ruin'd the Lodgment we had made upon the Gorge

Fourneau The Chamber of a Mine, being a Hollow made under some Work that is to be blown up, the Top of it sometimes made like a Priest's Cap, that is, with four or five Hollows in it, that the

the Powder may find the more Passage. Sometimes this Chamber is 5 or 6 Foot every way, being exactly Square, which is most usual. About a Thousand Weight of Powder, either in Bags or Barrels, is the common Charge of one of these Chambers; but it is at the Discretion of the Engineer to add or diminish this Proportion, according to the Bulk or Nature of the Soil he is to blow up, whether loose Earth, or Rock. For sometimes they make four or five Chambers under one Work, each of which has not above an Hundred Weight of Powder.

Fourneau Superficial. Vide *Caisson.*

Fraises. Stakes about six or seven Foot long, whereof about One third Part is drove into the Wall of a fortify'd Place, a little below the *Cordon* of the Wall, and in such Places as are not fac'd or lin'd with Wall, they are planted on the Outside of the Rampart, about the Foot of the Parapet. They are always stuck sloaping a little, that is, not quite Parallel to the Level of the Plain, but the Points hanging down a little, that Men may not stand on them. They serve to prevent Scalades and Desertion.

To Fraize a Batalion, is so to line it every way with Pikes, that it may stand the Shock of a Body of Horse.

Front. The foremost Rank of a Batalion, Squadron, or other Body of Men. To Front every way, is when the Men are fac'd to all Sides.

To

The Front of a Plac, which is also call'd e *Tenaille*, and the Face of a Place, is at Part that is contain'd betwixt the oints of any two neighbouring Bastions, at is, the Curtin, the two Flanks and e two Faces of the Bastions that face e another

d Fuze A Pipe full of Wild-fire put to the Touch-hole of a Bomb, Grana- or the like, to fire it.

Fuzileers Foot Soldiers arm'd with relocks, which are generally slung here is a Regiment of *Fuzileers* for the uard of the Artillery

G

G*Abions*, or *Cannon Baskets* Great Baskets 5 or 6 Foot high, and a- ut four Foot Diameter, as well at the ttom as the Top These are fill'd with rth, and serve to cover Men against the emies Fire, either as Merlons on Bat- ies, planting Guns between them, or make Lodgments upon any Posts, or e to serve as Parapets to the Ap- paches, when the Attack is carry'd on ng a Stony or Rocky Way

Ga ry A Passage made a-cross the tch of a Town besieg'd, with Timbers en'd on the Ground, and plank'd over, Planks all loaded with Earth to secure Miners from the Enemies Fire, and Galery itself secur'd against Fire by Earth on it The Word *Galery* is al- us'd for the Branch of a Mine, that is, arrow Passage under Ground, leading

to

to the Mine that is carry'd on under Work design'd to be blown up W drove the Enemy from our *Galery* w Hand-Granadoes The Besieg'd and I siegers carry'd on their *Galeries* und Ground, which often met, and were stroy'd, or became useless

Garrison This Word signifies eit the Place into which Forces are put in Winter-Quarters, or the Troops the selves put into a fortify'd Place to fend it, being strong Holds, as are ge rally along Frontiers

Gate Made of strong Planks with Ir Bars to oppose an Enemy The Gate a strong Hold ought to be in the mid of a Curtin, that it may be well defend by the Flanks and Faces Those which in the Flank weaken the most necess Part of the Fortification, and when th are in the Face, they are still more pre dicial to the Bastion, which ought to l clear to make Retrenchments upon oc sion

Gazons Sods or Turfs, cut square l large Bricks, cover'd with Grass and us to face the Outsides of Works made Earth, to keep it up, and prevent its mo dring The common Length of a *Gaz* about a Foot its Breadth about half a Fo and the same Thickness *Traverses* made pass a Ditch, are often cover'd with *Gaz* laid on Planks to save them from Fire

Gendarmes, or Men at Arms Hor men who formerly fought in compl rmour ; now a select Body of Horse in ance, being in all 9 Independent roops, not Regimented ; but commanded by Captains-Lieutenants, the ing being himself their Captain The roops of Life-Guards, those of the usketeers, and those of the Light-Horse the Queen, Dauphin, and Duke of leans, are reckon'd as *Gendarmes*, and ke Place as such

General of an Army He that commands it in Chief, who, to be fit for so eat an Employ, ought to rely more on s Conduct than Strength, to be well ill'd in the Art of attacking strong aces, and know how to encamp so advangeously, that it may be in his Choice hether he will fight or not, so that his isdom may gain the Love and Affection his Troops, make them confide in n, and be a Terror to his Enemies. here are also Lieutenant-Generals, Ma-r-Generals, Colonel-Generals, Commissy-Generals, and Quartermaster-Genes of which we shall speak under their rticular Letters

General The Beat of Drum so call'd, the first which gives notice, commonin the Morning early, for the Foot to in a readiness to march

General Officers Vide *Officer*

Gin An Engine for lifting or raising Great Guns

To give Ground To retire, to lose the t a Body of Men is in

Glacis This Word in general signifies a very easy little Slope, which distin guishes it from the *Talus* For in th *Glacis*, the Height is always less than th Base of the Slope , but in the *Talus* th Height is equal to, or more than th Base of the Slope. The Name of *Glaci* is particularly apply'd to the Slope of th Parapet of the *Covert-way*, which falls of even with the Level of the Field Th *Glacis* is also call'd *Esplanade* , but th Word in this Sense grows out of Date When the Trenches are brought within . Paces of the *Glacis*, there is no approachin nearer the *Covert-way* but by *Sappe*, to pro ceed according to the Rules of Art, unle they resolve to carry the Counterscarp b Assault

Gorge The Entrance that leads into th Body of a Work, as *I M Fig* 1 All *Gorges* mu be plain without any Parapet, lest whe the Besiegers have possess'd themselves the Work, that Parapet should cover th from the Fire of the Place , but the G ges are Palisado'd to prevent Surpri and during the Siege they generally m little Mines, Coffers, and *Fourneaux* und them to blow up the Enemies before th can lodge themselves The several Gorg are distinguish'd as follows

The Gorge of a Bastion It is form'd two Lines, drawn both ways from t Angle of the *Polygon* to the Angles of t Curtin or Flank

The Gorge of a Plat Bastion, Is a straight Line reaching between the two Flanks.

The Gorge of a Half-Moon, or *Ravelin*; is the Space between the two Ends of their Faces next the Place.

The Gorge of other Out-works, is the interval betwixt their Sides next the Ditch.

Governor of a Garrison. A considerable Officer representing the King's Person, whose Authority extends not only over the Inhabitants and Garrison, but over all Troops that may be there in Winter-Quarters, or Quarters of Refreshment.

Granadeers. Soldiers arm'd with a good Sword, a Hatchet, a Fire-lock flung, and a Pouch full of Hand-Granadoes. Every Batalion of Foot, of late Years, has generally a Company of Granadeers belonging to it, or else four or five Granadeers belong to each Company of the Batalion, and upon occasion form a Company of themselves. There are Horse and Foot Granadeers, and they have often been found very serviceable.

Granadoes. Are small Shells, concave Globes, or hollow Balls, some made of Iron, some of Tin, others of Wood, and even of Pastboard, but most commonly of Iron, because the Splinters of it do most Execution. This Globe or Hollow is fill'd with fine Powder, and into the Touch hole of it is stuck a Fuzé of Powder, beaten and temper'd with Charcoal Dust, that it may not flash but burn gently till it comes to the Charge. These are thrown by hand into Places where Men stand thick, and particularly into Trenches and Lodgments the Enemy makes, and are of good use

Great Guns Vide *Cannon*.

Guard The Duty perform'd by a Body of Men with Watchfulness, to secure all against the Attempts and Surprizes of an Enemy To be upon Guard, To Mount the Guard, To Relieve the Guard, The Officer of the Guard, The Sergeant of the Guard In time of Danger all Guards are drawn by Lot, to prevent any treacherous Officers having the opportunity of betraying a Post to the Enemy Troops in Garrison generally mount the Guard every third Night, and have two Nights to rest

The Main Guard In Garrison, is that to which all less Guards are subordinate, the commanding Officer keeping it with the greater Number of Men In the Field it is a considerable Body of Horse detach'd to the Head of the Camp, to secure the Army by keeping a Watchful Eye upon all the Avenues that lead to it

Advanc'd Guard A Party of 15 or [illegible] Horse, commanded by a Lieutenant, beyond, but within Sight of the Main Guard for the greater Security of the Camp

Guards du Corps, or *Life-Guards* The Troops of Horse-Guards maintain'd for the Security of the King's Person, which take Place of all other Troops of Horse

Regiments of Guards Regiments of Foot doing Duty wheresoever the King's Person is on is for his Defence, with Precedence before all other Regiments of Foot

Picket, or *Piquet Guards* Small Guards commanded by Lieutenants or Ensigns at the Head of every Regiment, as they are encamp'd, to be always in readiness against all Surprizes

Guerite A Sentinel's Box, being like a little Tower made either of Stone, Brick or Wood, to preserve the Sentinel from ill-Weather Some call them *Echaugettes* They are generally plac'd on the Points of Bastions and Angles of the *Epaul*, and sometimes in the middle of a Curtin, and are to hang a little over the Wall, that the Sentinel may look down to the Foot of the Ramparts

Guidon An Officer to carry the Standard in the Troops of Guards The same Word is also taken for the Standard it self

Guns Vide *Cannon*

H

HAlf-Files The three foremost Men in the Field, when a Battalion is drawn up, are call'd the *Front Half Files*, and the three hindmost Men the *Rear Half Files*

Half-Moon An Out work consisting of two Faces, which makes an *Angle Saillant*, the Gorge whereof bends in like a Bow or Crescent, and is ever us'd to cover the Point of a Bastion, which distinguishes them from *Ravelins*, always plac'd before

 the

the Curtin, but they are defective, as being ill flank'd At present only Engineers distinguish between *Ravelins* and *Half-Moons*, for the Soldiers and other Persons call them all indifferently *Half-Moons*, tho' improperly, yet Custom prevails, especially because the Difference is rather in the Situation, than in the Thing it self. Vide *Ravelin*

To Halt, Is to discontinue the March of Troops, to stand still, to stop in order to rest, or on any other Account whatsoever, and so the Word of Command for Men to stop, when they are marching, is *Halt*

Hay, Is a straight Rank of Men drawn up exactly in a Line

Head of the Camp The Ground before the Camp, where the *Biovac*, or on which the Army draws out.

Head of a Work The Front of it next the Enemy, and farthest from the Body of the Place

Hedges To Line Hedges Vide *Line*

Height Vide *Eminence*

Hendecagon A Figure that has eleven Sides, and as many Angles, capable of being fortify'd with the like Number of Bastions

Heptagon A Figure that has seven Sides and Angles, each capable of a Regular Bastion

Herisson A Barrier made of only one Piece of Wood stuck thick with abundance of Iron Spikes, born up and equally balanc'd in the Middle on a Stake

bo

bout which it turns, to open or shut the Passage in the Nature of a Turn-stile

Herse Vide *Portcullis*

Herse, Is also a Harrow, the Besieg'd for want of *Chevaux de Frize*, lay in the Way, or on Breaches with the Points up, to hinder the March of Horse and Foot

Hersillon A Plank 10 or 12 Foot long, stuck full of Nails with the Points up, for the same Use as the Herse

Hexagon A Figure that has six equal Sides, and as many Angles, each capable of a Regular Bastion

Hogsheads, fill'd with Earth They serve to make Parapets to cover the Men, instead of *Gabions* and *Earth-Bags*

Hollow Square Vide *Square*

Hony-Comb in Cannon Flaws in the Metal, a Fault in Casting, and dangerous in Firing

Horizontal Superficies. The plain Field lying upon a Level without any rising or falling

Horn-work, In French, *Ouvrage a Corne*; Is an Out-work, the Head whereof is fortify'd by two *Demi-Bastions*, or *Epaulments*, joyn'd by a Curtin, and clos'd by Parallel Sides, terminating at the Gorge of the Work

Horse, is taken for that Body of Men that serves a Horse-back So we say, a Body of Horse, the Horse fought well, the Horse march It is the same as *Cavalry*.

Horse de Frize. Vide *Chevaux de Frize*, and *Turnpikes*.

Horse-shooe A Round or Oval Work, enclos'd with a Parapet, rais'd in the Moat of a Marshy Place, or in low Grounds, or else to cover a Gate, and keep a *Corps de Garde* to prevent Surprizes

Hospital, Is a Place appointed for the Sick and Wounded Men, who have there a Number of Physicians, Surgeons and Servants, to attend and cure them

Hut The same as *Barack*. Vide *Barack*.

I.

ICHNOGRAPHY Vide *Plan*

To Incamp To pitch the Tents, or build Huts, on a Spot of Ground chosen for the Purpose, which is lodging an Army in the Field

Incampment The Lodging of an Army in the Field, according to its several Quarters, which are to lie conveniently for Water, Wood, and Forage, to be well posted to intrench, or at least have the Advantage of Ground, and so situated, that they may all face outwards At a Siege, the Place must be on their Backs, and the Foot are to cover the Horse, because they can be soonest at their Arms If the Enemy be near, the Cannon must be planted on the Side next him, and if the Camp be to march, the Cannon must be posted to face the Road they are to march

Indented Line Running in and out like the Teeth of a Saw, often us'd upon the Banks

Bank of a Counterscarp, upon a River, or Sea-side, and upon the Main Land, the Design that one Part may flank another.

Independent Company, or *Troop*. Vide *Company* and *Troop*.

Infantry The whole Body of Foot Soldiers, whether Independent Companies, or Regimented The Regiments of Foot Guards take Place of all others, the rest have Precedence according to Seniority This Precedence is for the eldest Regiment to march in the Front, the next in the Rear, and so on with the rest The eldest to incamp on the Right, the next on the Left, and so the rest in Course The Officers of Foot command those of Horse in Garrison, but are commanded by them in the Field

To Insult, or *To Assault* Is to attack a Post by open Force, coming on without any Shelter to fall to Handy strokes, without making use of Trenches, *Sappe*, or other Forms of Art, to gain Ground Foot by Foot The Counterscarp is generally insulted or assaulted, to prevent the Enemies having time to spring the *Fourneaux* or *Fougasses* they have prepar'd In these Attacks, the Granadeers commonly march at the Head of the other Troops, and there must be Pioneers ready to make a Lodgment to secure the Post gain'd

Intrench'd Any Post fortify'd with an Intrenchment

Intrenchment Any Work that fortifies a Post against the Enemies Attacks. It is generally taken for a Ditch or Trench, with a Parapet Intrenchments are also made of *Fascines* or *Faggots*, with Earth thrown over them, of *Gabions*, *Hogsheads*, or Bags fill'd with Earth, that cover the Men from the Enemies Fire

Invalide. A Soldier that has been maim'd in the Wars

To Invest a Place Is to secure all the Avenues, and distribute the Troops in the principal Posts, till the Artillery, and the rest of the Army, come up

Isosele Vide *Triangle*

L

LAdle for a Gun A long Staff with a Plate at the End of it, bow'd half round to put the Charge into the Piece

Lane To make a Lane To draw up Men in two Ranks facing one another, as on the Sides of a Street, or the like, for any great Person to pass through, or sometimes for a Soldier to run the Gauntlet

Lanspisade An Inferior Officer, subordinate to the Corporal, to assist him in his Duty, and supply his Place in Absence. In *France* he has some Allowance extraordinary, but not in *England* He is generally exempt from common Duty, except Rounds and Sentinels *Perdus* The true Name is *Anspesade*, but the *L* is added from the *French* Article *Le*

Lieutenant General A Great Commander, next in Place to the General of an

Army, who in Battle commands one of the Lines or Wings; a Detachment when they march, or a flying Camp, a Quarter at Siege, and one of the Attacks, when it is his Day of Duty

Lieutenant-General of the Artillery. The next to the General of the Artillery, who in his Absence has the whole Charge of all that belongs to it

Lieutenant du Roy. The Deputy Governor of all strong Towns in *France*, who is a Check upon the Governor, and commands in his Absence

Lieutenant-Colonel of Horse, Foot, or Dragoons The next in Post to the Colonel, and commands in his Absence The *French* have no Lieutenant-Colonels of Horse

Lieutenant of Horse, Foot, or Dragoons. The Officer of every Troop or Company next in Post to the Captain, and who commands in his Absence The *Spaniards* have no Lieutenants of Foot

Lieutenant Reform'd Vide *Reform'd.*

Lieutenant en Second Vide *Second.*

Life-Guards Vide *Guards de Corps.*

Light-Horse This Name is given to distinguish them from the Men at Arms formerly us'd, who were all in Armour, as now the *German Cuirassiers* In *England*, all are now call'd *Light-Horse*, except the Troops of Life-Guards In *France*, they except not only the *Guards de Corps*, but the two Troops of Musketeers a Horseback, and all the *Gendarmes*

Line, in the Geometrical Sense, sig-fies a Length without Breadth ; in the Art Military it is taken several Ways

Line, Is the drawing up of an Army for Battle, extending its Front as far as the Ground will allow, that it may not be flank'd The *Turkish* Armies often draw up in a crooked Line or Half-Moon, that, being very numerous, they may enclose their Enemies Christian Armies generally draw up in three Lines, the first, call'd the *Van*; the second, the *Main Body*, and the third, the *Reserve*, with a convenient Distance between them, and Intervals, that they may not put one another into Confusion

Line, in Fortification, bears several Significations In drawing a Plan upon Paper, it is only a plain Line drawn from one Point to another. On the Ground, it is sometimes taken for a Trench with a Parapet, and sometimes for a Row of Gabions, or Bags full of Earth, to cover Men from the Enemies Fire So we say, when the Trenches were carry'd on within 30 Paces of the Glacis, we drew two Lines, one on the Right, and the other on the Left, for a Place of Arms

Line of Defence A Line that represents the Flight of a Ball; but particularly a Musket Ball, from the Place where the Musketeer must stand, to scour the Face of the Bastion There are two sorts of this Line, the *Fichant*, and the *Razant* or *Flanking*

ine of Defence fix'd, or *Fichant*; Is a
e drawn from the Angle of the Cur-
to the Point of the opposite Bastion,
ich is not to exceed 800 Foot; or, as
French say, 120 *Toises*, because that is
length of the Port of a Musket, and
n that Point of the Curtin and Flank,
Face of the opposite Bastion is to be
ended, as *M P Fig* 1

ine Razant, Stringent or *Flanking*, or
d Flank A Line drawn from the
nt of the Bastion along the Face, till
omes to the Curtin, which shews
much of the Curtin will clear or
r the Face, as *N P Fig* 1

ine forming the Flank A Line drawn
n the Angle, form'd by the two De-
Gorges of the Bastion, to the Angle
he Flank This only us'd by *Dutch*
ineers

pital Line. A Line drawn from the
t of the Bastion, to the Point where
two Demi-Gorges meet.

ines of Circumvallation, and *Contraval-*
n Vide *Circumvallation*, and *Contra-*
a ion

ines of Communication Are Trenches
run from one Work to another, so that
may pass between them without be-
expos'd to the Enemy; therefore the
le Intrenchment round any Place is
etimes called a Line of Communica-
, because it leads to all the Works.

ines of Approaches Vide *Approaches*.

ine. Vide *Cordeau*.

To

To Line Hedges To plant Muske along them under their Covert; to upon an Enemy that comes open, or defend them from the Horse

Links of Dragoon or Granadeer H ses; are distinct Reins or Thongs of ther, made fast to the Horses Bri with which Dragoons and Granad when they dismount, link or make their Horses one to another, that may not disperse, every tenth Man ing left a Horse back to look to them.

Lizier Vide *Foreland*

Lock of a Gun; is all that Part w belongs to the firing of it, and con the Cock, the Pan, &c

Lockspit The small Cut or Tr made with the Spade, to mark out first Lines of a Work that is to be m

Lodgment, Is a Work made up dangerous Post in carrying on a S as on the *Covert-way*, the Out-works, Breach, in a Ditch, or any other gain'd from the Besieged, to cover Men from their Fire, either by ca up Earth, by *Gabions* or Bags ful Earth, Palisades, Wooll-packs, Fasc Mantelets, or any other thing that cover Soldiers in the Place they gain'd, and resolve to keep.

Lozange Vide *Rhombus*

Lunette A small Work, *Counterg* or *Envelope*, made in the Ditch before Curtin It consists of two Faces, mak an Angle inwards, and are gener

ma

ade in Ditches full of Water, to serve ſtead of a *Fausse-Braye*, and dispute the ſſage of the Ditch The *Terre-plain* it is rais'd but a little above the ſur- ce of the Water, and is but 12 Foot oad, with a Parapet three Fathom ick, ſo that the whole breadth of the *nette* is five Fathom Vide *Counterguard*, d *Envelope*

M

MAdrier A thick Plank, generally us'd to cover the Mouth of a Pe- d when it is Charg'd, and apply'd th it to the Gates, or other Places, to torn or broke up There are alſo *arie s* made of longer Planks than thoſe r the Petards, which are cover'd with n, and loaded with Earth to ſave em from Fire. The Pioneers lay them er the *Sappes*, or Lodgments, where ere is need of being cover'd over-head. ſtead of them, they ſometimes uſe ays

Main-Battle Vide *Battle*

Main Guard Vide *Guard*

Major There are ſeveral ſorts of Ma- rs, all conſiderable Officers, and that ght to be Men of Experience They e, a Major-General, a Major of a Bri- de, a Major of Horſe or Foot, and a own-Major

Major-General An Officer that receives e General's Orders, and delivers them

out

out to the Majors of Brigades, with whom he resolves what Troops are to mount Guards, to go out upon Parties, form Detachments, or be sent on Convoys. He also views the Ground to incamp, and performs several other Duties, being subordinate to the General and Lieutenant-General, and the next Supreme Commanding Officer to them

Major of a Brigade, either of Horse, or Foot, receives Orders, and the Word from the Major-General, and gives them to the Major of each Regiment

Major of a Regiment of Horse, Foot, or Dragoons; Is to convey all Orders to the Regiment to draw it up, and exercise it, to see it march in good Order, to look to its Quarters, to Rally it if broken, &c. and is the only Officer among the Foot that is a Horse-back in time of Service, to be every where as occasion requires

Town-Major The third Officer in order in a Garrison, and next to the Deputy-Governor He ought to understand Fortification, and has a particular Charge of the Guards, Rounds, Patrouilles and Sentinels

Mantelets Blinds made of thick Planks Musket-proof, and often cover'd with Tin, which the Pioneers generally roll before them, they being fix'd upon Wheels, to cover them from the Enemies Fire There are double *Mantlets*, which make an Angle, and stand Square to form two Fronts, and cover the Front and nd Flank. These have double Planks, ith Earth ramm'd in between them. They must be five Foot high, and Three breadth They are sometimes the ickness of two or three Planks, bound gether with Iron Plates.

A March; Is either the moving of a ody of Men, or the Beat of Drum us d hen Soldiers are upon March

To March, Is for a Body of Men to ove from one Place to another

Mareschal de Bataille It was once a dinct Command ; but this Duty being ly part of the Major-General's, it is w executed by him

Mareschal de Camp. A General Officer xt in Post to the Lieutenant-General, d I find no difference betwixt him and e Major-General.

Master de Camp; Is no other than a Conel of Horse, so call'd in *France* and *in*, where they give the Title of Conels only to those that command Rements of Foot and Dragoons, whereas th us, they are all indifferently call'd lonels

Master de Camp General The Second neral Officer over all the Regiments of ght-Horse, and next to the Colonelneral He has a Regiment of Horse onging to him, which takes the Second st of Honour next to the Colonel-Geral's This in *France*, for there is no h in the *English* Forces

Match A sort of Rope made on purpose,

pose, which once lighted at the En
burns on gradually and regularly, witho
ever going out as long as any of it
left It is us'd for firing of Match-Lo
Muskets, and all sorts of Great Guns,
is also laid in Mines that are to blow
so many Hours after, and the Time is
gulated by the Length of Match there
to burn before the fire comes to
Powder, and by the same Rule, th
that are us'd to it, know how the Ho
pass

Match-Lock, is a Musket that is fi
with a Match fix'd on the Cock open
the Pan, now much out of use, Fi
Locks being altogether prefer'd bef
them.

Maxims in Fortification. Are cer
general Rules establish'd by Engine
and grounded on Reason and Exp
ence, which being well observ'd, a Pl
fortify'd to them will be in a good
sture of Defence The chief of them
these that follow

1. *There must be no part of the Fortifi.ti
but what is discover'd and flank'd by th
sieged:* Because if any part were under
vert, it would be the more easily
tack'd, as having no Defence from
Place

2 *The Place fortify'd must Comman
Parts round about it* Lest the Enemy h
the opportunity of concealing their
signs, make their Approaches under
vert, or over-look and batter the Plac

3 *The Works farthest remov'd from the* [C]*enter of the Place must ever be open, and* [co]*mmanded by the nearest* That the Ene[m]y may be expos'd to the Besieged, when [the]y have made themselves Masters of [an]y of them

4 *The Flank'd Angle, or the Point of the* [B]*astion, must be of 70 Degrees at least*, That [it] may be the stronger to withstand the [E]nemy's Battery

5 *The Acute Flank'd Angle, the nearer it* [is] *to a Right Angle, is the better* The [F]lank'd Angle, that is, a Right Angle, is [c]ertainly the firmest against the Enemies [B]atteries

6. *The shortest Faces are the best*, Because [th]e long Ones are the weaker, the Enemy [h]aving the more Front to attack them [H]owever, they must be at least 40 or 50 [F]athom long, to be able to defend the [O]ut-works.

7 *The Flank must have some part under* [C]*overt* That is, it must be cover'd by an [O]rillon, otherwise its Defences are soon [r]uin'd, and as soon as the Enemy is lodg[e]d in the Counterscarp, the Place must [C]apitulate

8. *There must be a perfect Agreement be*[t]*ween all the Maxims of Fortification to render* [i]*t perfect* That is, such Care must be [ta]ken, that the adhering too strongly to [o]ne, does not prejudice another

Merlon That part of the Parapet which [i]s between two *Embrazures* of a Battery. [T]he length of a *Merlon* is generally nine Foot

Foot next the Guns, and ſix on the ou ſide Its Height 6 Foot, and its Thick neſs 18.

Military Execution The ravaging an deſtroying of a Country that refuſes t pay Contribution

Mine A Hole dug in a Wall, or un der Ground, and carry'd on like a Pa ſage or Alley, about four Foot ſquare with ſeveral Turnings and Windings it At the End of them, that is under t Place deſign'd to be blown up, is th Chamber of the Mine The further it is carry'd, the more Danger it is in being diſappointed by the Enemy, that it is beſt not to carry it too far, an to make a ſecond where the firſt has take effect Vide *Fourneau*, *Galery*, and *Pu* or *Well*, *Coffers* and *Foucades*

Miners Men appointed to work i the Mines, being a particular Compan of themſelves, commanded by a Captai of the Regiment of *Fuziliers*, which Re giment is appointed for the Service o the Artillery When the Miner is work, he wears a ſort of Hood, to kee the Earth, that falls, out of his Eyes

Minion Ordnance A ſmall Gun 3 Inche Diameter in the Bore, 7 Foot long weighing about 800 Pounds, takes Charge of 2 Pounds 8 Ounces of Pow der, and carries a Bullet 2 Inches 7 Eight Diameter, and 3 Pounds 4 Ounce Weight. Its Shot point-blank 120 Pace

Minion, of the longest Size, Is 3 Inches Eights in the Bore, 8 Foot long, ighs 1000 Pounds Its Charge, 3 Pounds Ounces of Powder, and carries a Bul- 3 Inches Diameter, and weighing ounds 12 Ounces Its Shot point-blank , Paces

Moat, Ditch or *Fosse* A Depth or Trench round a Town or Fortress; which ng under the Fire of the Rampaits, st therefore be allso well Flank'd The adth and Depth of it is more or less ording to the nature of the Earth, ac- ding to which the Slope of the Scarp Counterscarp is also regulated In eral, it ought to be so wide, that no e or Ladder can be laid over it, that from 16 to 22 Fathom, and between and 16 Foot deep Wet Ditches are ays shallower than the Dry, but the are counted the best If the Ditch dry, or has but little Water, there is nmonly another small Trench cut e round along the middle of it

Moineau Some give this Name to a le Plat-Bastion, rais'd before a Curtin is too long, and has two other Ba- ns at the Ends, which being beyond sket-shot one of another, must be nded by this Plat-Bastion Sometimes oyns to the Curtin, and sometimes is ded by a Moat

Mont Pagnote, or *Post of the Invulnerable*. Eminence chosen out of Cannon-shot he Place besieg'd, where curious Per-

sons

sons post themselves, to see an Arm and the Manner of the Siege, out of Da ger

Mortar-Peice. A very short Gun, wi an extraordinary large Bore, and a ch Chamber, this to hold the Charge Powder, the other to contain the Bo it is to throw These Mortars are alw mounted on low Carriages, like th us'd at Sea, the Wheels being each one Piece They are not fir'd right f ward, like Cannon, but mounted into Air, so that the Bomb ascending a Heighth, falls with the greater Fo and flies the further Sometimes Mortars are charg'd with Baskets full Stones, which they throw into Tow and do great Execution, bacause fall thick, there is no Place of Safety fr them

Motions of an Army The several M ches and Countermarches it makes, changing of its Posts, either for be Ground, to force an Enemy to Ba to avoid it, or the like

Mount Vide *Cavalier*

To Mount. To mount the Guard, m on that Duty To mount a Breach run up it in an Assault

To Mount the Trenches Vide *Trench*

Musk.t The most convenient commonest Sort of Fire-Arm that is in War Generally two thirds of e Company, and consequently of every giment of Foot, are arm'd with th the rest with Pikes They are to ry a Ball of about an Ounce Weight, all to be made to the same Bore, lest y should prove useless by not fitting Bullet. The Length of the Line of ence is settl'd by the Distance a Mus- will carry to do Execution, which is nted about 240 Yards, and accord- ly all the Works are proportion'd

Musket Baskets These are about a Foot, Foot and half high, 8 or 10 Inches meter at bottom, and a Foot at the , so that being fill'd with Earth, there oom to lay a Musket between them bottom, being set on low Brest-works Parapets, or upon such as are beaten vn

Musketeers. The Soldiers in every Re- nent of Foot that are arm'd with Mus- s In *France*, there are two Compa- s, or rather Troops, call *Mousquetaires Roy*, or the King's Musketeers, com- 'd all of Gentlemen excellently well unted, who serve either a Foot or a rse-back, and signalize themselves up- all desperate Occasions, being there y for Preferment The King him- f is their Captain, and the Officer com- nding each of them is call'd *Captain- utenant*, yet each of them commands Colonel both of Horse and Foot, and cordingly takes Place of all younger lonels of either They are reckon'd *Gendarmes*, and march next to the *Scotch ndarmes*

Mus-

Musketoon A short Fire-Arm, with very large Bore to carry several Musk or Pistol Bullets, proper to fire amon a Crowd, or to keep a Pass. It is the sa as a Blunderbuss.

Muster A Review of Troops to ta an Account of their Numbers, and th Condition they are in, viewing th Arms and Accoutrements, and accor ing to the Number that appears, t Pay for them is deliver'd to their Of cers

Mustermaster-General. Vide *Commissa General of Musters.*

Muster Rolls The Rolls or Lists Soldiers found in each Company, Troo and Regiment, by which they are pa and the Strength of the Army is know

Muzzle ; Is the Mouth of any Pie at which it is loaded and discharg'd

Muzzle-Ring of a Gun That wh encompasses and strengthens the Muz or Mouth of a Cannon.

N.

TO *Nail Cannon*, or, as some call *To Cloy* To drive a large Spi by main Force into the Touch-hole o Gun ; or for want of Spikes, small Fli or other Stones. This renders the Ca non unserviceable, either stopping up t Touch-hole, or, if the Spike be taken o leaving it so large that it cannot be fir because it takes too much Vent the

T

The Remedy is, to drill a new Touch-hole. The most honourable Thing the Garrison of a Place besieg'd can propose to it self in a Sally, is to Nail up the Enemies Cannon. Some call it, To Cloy, as was said at first, but this is an antiquated Word.

O

OCtogon. A Figure that has eight Sides, and as many Angles, capable of being fortify'd with the like number of Bastions.

Officer, in general, signifies a Person that has some Command in the Body he serves in. But more strictly it is taken only for those that have Commissions, so it includes all from the General to the Corporal in the largest Sense, and in the strictest from the General to the Ensign or Cornet, for which Reason Officers are thus distinguish'd.

General Officers. Those that have Power not only over one Regiment, Troop, or Company; but in general, over a Body compos'd of several Regiments. These are the General, Lieutenant-General, Major-General, Brigadier-General, Colonel, Quarter-Master and Adjutant-General.

Field-Officers. Those that have a Power and Command over a whole Regiment; and not only over one single Troop, or Company, which are the Colonel, Lieutenant-Colonel, and Major: So cal-

led, because they appear most at the[ir]
Command when the Regiment draws o[ut]
into the Field; for not being subject t[o]
common Duty of Mounting Guards in
Quarters, they are not there so much seen.

Commission-Officers All those that ha[ve]
the King's Commission, which are all from
the General to the Ensign and Cornet in-
clusive

Subaltern-Officers The Lieutenant, Ensign, and Cornet of Horse, Foot and
Dragoons, are so call'd

Warrant, and Staff-Officers. Those wh[o]
have not the King's Commission, but are
appointed by the Colonels and Captains
as Quarter-masters, Serjeants, Corporals
and in the same Number are includ[ed]
Chaplains and Surgeons

To open the Trenches The first breaking
of Ground made by the Besiegers, in orde[r]
to the carrying on their Approaches towards the Place besieg'd

Order of Battle The placing of the Ba[t]-
talions and Squadrons in one Line or more
according as the Ground will allow, t[o]
ingage the Enemy to the best Advantag[e]

Orders, in general, signify all that i[s]
commanded by Superiors, and is sometimes taken only for the Word

Order your Arms; Is to place the Bu[tt]
End of the Musket on the Ground, clo[se]
to the right Foot, with the right Hand under the Muzzle The Pike is order'd i[n]
the same manner, holding it with th[e]
right Hand the Height of the Should[er]

Or-

Ordnance. Vide *Cannon*.

Orgues. Long and substantial Pieces of Wood, every one separate from the other, hanging with Ropes over the Gateway of a City perpendicularly, and ready upon any Surprise attempted by an Enemy, to be let drop down in the Gateway to stop it up, without being subject to the Danger that the Enemy may clap any Piece or Wooden Horse a-cross the Gate, and so keep up the whole Range of Pieces as may happen with *Portcullisses*, because the Pieces they consist of being all made fast to one another, when one stops all stop; whereas the *Orgues* being also sever'd from one another, the stopping of one is no hindrance to the fall of the rest, and therefore the *Orgues* are esteem'd better than *Portcullisses*.

Orillon, or *Blind*. A Mass of Earth fac'd with Wall, advancing beyond the *Epaul*, or Shoulder of Bastions that have *Cazemattes* to cover the Cannon in them, and prevent its being dismounted by the Enemy. Some *Orillons* are round, and others almost square, call'd *Epaulments*.

Orthographical Section, or *Profile*, is that draught which shews the thickness, breadth, depth, and height of any Work, as it would appear if perpendicularly cut off from the highest to the lowest Part of it. It does not represent the length of the Work, which the *Plan* does, but then the *Plan* does not shew the height and depth, but represents the breadth, *Fig.* 2.

Explanation of *Fig.* 2.

1,	10	*The Level of the Plain*
1,	2	*The Base of the Rampart*
2,	5	*The Fausse Braye*
3,	4	*The Space of the Fausse-Bray*
4,	5	*The Base of the Parapet of Fausse-Braye*
5,	6	*The Berme or Foreland*
6,	7	*The Breadth of the Ditch*
7,	9	*The Covert way*
9,	10	*The Glacis*
3,	4	*The Breadth of the Banquet of Fausse-Braye*
8,	9	*The Breadth of the Banquet of Covert-way*
1,	19	2, 26. *The Height of the Ramp*
19,	20	*The inward Talus of the Ramp*
26,	30	*The outward Talus of the Ram*
22,	30	*The Base of the Parapet*
22,	23.	*The Height of the Parapet*
23	25	*The Glacis of the Parapet*
2[illegible],	0	*The Height of the Banquet*
24.	0	*The Height above the Banquet*
4,	27	*The Height of the Banquet of Fausse-Braye*
27,	28	*The Glacis of the Fausse Braye*
5,	11	*The Depth of the Ditch*
11,	12	*The Talus of the Ditch*
6,	12	*The Escarp*
7	15	*The Counterscarp*
13,	14	*The Breadth of the Cuvette*
13,	17	*The Depth of the Cuvette*
17	18	*The Talus of the Cuvette*
7	29	*The Depth of the Covert-way*
[illegible]	21	*The Terre-plain of the Rampart*

[Fig. 2.]

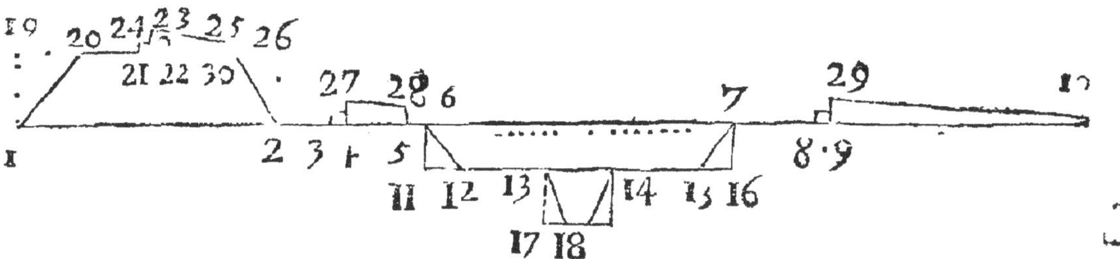

Out-works. All the Works that cove the Body of a Place next the Campaign as *Ravelins*, *Half-Moons*, *Horn-Works*, *Tenailles*, *Crown-works*, *Swallow's-Tails*, *Envelopes*, and the like It is a general Rule That if there be several *Out-works* one before another, to cover one and the same *Tenaille* of a Place, those that are nearest the Place must gradually, one after another, command those that are farthest advanc'd out into the Campaign, that is must have higher Ramparts, that they may over-look and fire upon the Besiegers when they have possess'd themselves of the farthest The Gorges of them must be always plain, for fear, if they had any Parapet, it might serve the Besiegers when they are Masters of it, to cover themselves against the Fire of the Besieg'd; and therefore the Gorges are only Palisado'd to prevent Surprise.

Oxygon Vide *Triangle*.

P

PAce A Measure us'd in Fortification and much spoke of in Military Discipline There is a Common and a Geometrical *Pace* The Common *Pace* is generally counted a Yard, the Geometrical 5 Foot An *Italian* Mile is 1000 Geometrical *Paces*, and three of these Miles a *French* League

Palisades, *Palisadoes*, or *Piles* Great Wooden Stakes, or Spars, 6 or 7 Inches

Squar

Square, and 8 Foot long, whereof 3 Foot are let into the Ground They are planted on the Avenues of all Places that may be carry'd by Assault, and even by regular Attack Some Palisades are drove down-right into the Ground, others make an Angle, bowing down a little towards the Ground next the Enemy, that if they should throw Cords about them to pull them up, they may slip off Palisades are planted on the *Berme*, or *Foreland* of Bastions, and at the Gorges of Half-Moons, and other Out-works The Bottom of the Ditch is also palisado'd, but above all the Parapet of the *Covert-way* Some place the Palisadoes three Foot from the said Parapet outwards to the Campaign; but of late they have been planted in the middle of the *Covert-way* They are to stand so close, that no Interval remain between them, but what will serve for the Muzzle of a Musket, or to thrust a Pike through Palisades are either pull'd up shaking them with Ropes, cut down by the Granadeers, beaten down with Cannon, or burnt down with tarr'd Fascines or Faggots

Pan The same as the Face of a Bastion Vide *Face*

Pan The Pan, in Fire-Arms is a small Iron Cavity, sticking to the Barrel, next to the Chamber, to contain as much Powder as will take Fire without, and convey it through the Touch-hole to the Charge within

Parade The Place where Troops assemble or draw together, in order to Mount Guards, or for any Service

Parallel Tho' this be properly a Term in Geometry, yet being often us'd in Fortification, it deserves to be explain'd Parallel Lines, are those which are of an equal Distance from one another in every Part of them, and will so continue, tho' never so far extended, so that they can never meet, or draw nearer The opposite Sides of a Square, are parallel to one another The Ranks of a Batalion are parallel, and so are the Files The Counterscarp is drawn parallel to the Face of its Bastion, and generally the Line of Approaches is drawn Parallel to the Face of the Place attack'd, to prevent its being *Enfiladed*, or Scour'd in length

Parapet, or *Breast-work* A Work rais'd to cover Men against the Enemies Cannon, and Small-Shot, on Ramparts, Bastions, *&c* and must be made of Earth, and not of Stones, lest they, being beaten to pieces, do Mischief It is eighteen or twenty Foot thick, six Foot high towards the Place, and four or five towards the Campaign, which Difference of Height makes the Glacis, or Slope for the Musketeers to fire down into the Ditch, or at least upon the Counterscarp The Name of Parapet, is given in general to any Line that covers Men from the Enemies Fire, so there are Parapets of Barrels, of Gabions, and of Bags fill'd with Earth

Park of the Artillery A Post in the Camp, out of Cannon-Shot of the Enemy, and fortify'd to secure the Magazines and Ammunition, where, to prevent Accidents of Fire, only Pikemen do Duty Every Attack at a Siege, has its *Park of Artillery*

Park of Provisions A Place appointed in the Rear of every Regiment, for Sutlers and others to bring Things to sell to furnish the Army

Parley To beat or sound a *Parley* Vide *Chamade*

Partisan A good Partisan is an able cunning Soldier, well skill'd in commanding a Party, who knows the Country, and how to avoid Ambushes, and surprize the Enemy

Partisan or *Pertuisan.* A Weapon not unlike a Halbert, us'd sometimes by Lieutenants of Foot.

Party A small Body of Horse or Foot sent out to discover, or upon any Military Execution The King of *France*, to prevent Robberies, has order'd, That all Parties of Enemies, under 15 in Number, that do not produce an Order under a Commanding Officer's Hand, if taken, be sent to the Gallies as Robbers

Pas de Souris Vide *Forclana*

Pasi-Volans Vide *Faggots.*

Pate A Platform, like that they call a Horse-shoe, not always regular, but for the most part oval, encompass'd with a Parapet, without any other Defence for the most part, except only that fore-right, and having nothing to flank it They are commonly erected in Marshy Grounds to cover a Gate of a Town

Patrouille A Round going about in the Night, consisting generally of five or six Men commanded by a Serjeant, (or of fewer, if Horse) that set out from the *Corps de Garde*, to see what is done in the Streets, and keep Peace and Quietness in the Town

Pay Is the Wages given to a Soldier for his Maintenance in his Prince's Service, and is greater or less, according to the Custom of several Countries

Pay-Master, Is he who is intrusted with the Money, and has the Charge of paying the Soldiers

Pedrero A small sort of Cannon, most used aboard Ships, to fire Stone or broken Iron upon Boarding Some of them are made to open at the Breech, to take in the Charge that way

Peloton Vide *Platoon*

Pentagon A Figure of five Sides, and as many Angles, capable of being fortify'd with the same number of Bastions

Perpendicular A right Line, falling from, or lifting it self upon another upright, without inclining one way or the other, and making the Angles on both Sides equal

Petard An Engine of Metal, almost in the Shape of a Hat, about 7 Inches deep, and about 5 Inches over at the Mouth

When

When charg'd with fine Powder well beaten, it is cover'd with a *Madrier*, or Plank, bound down fast with Ropes running through Handles which are round the Rim near the Mouth of it This *Petard* is applied to Gates or Barriers of such Places as are design'd to be surpriz'd, to blow them up They are also us'd in Counter-Mines to break through into the Enemies Galeries, and disappoint their Mines

Pickaxes Us'd in digging Ground when too hard for the Spade, but too common to require more to be said of them, tho' mention'd as being a Tool very necessary in an Army

Picket, or *Piquet-Guard* Vide *Guard*

Picket or *Piquet*, Is a Stake sharp at the End, which serves to mark out the Ground and Angles of a Fortification, when the Engineer is laying down the *Plan* They are commonly pointed with Iron There are also large *Piquets*, which are drove into the Earth, to hold together the *Fascines* or *Faggots*, in any Work cast up in haste *Pickets* are also Stakes drove into the Ground, by the Tents of the the Horse in the Field to tie their Horses to, and before the Foot to rest their Arms about them in a Ring, each Company has commonly three, two for Muskets, and one for Pikes Horsemen that have committed any considerable Offence, are sentenc'd to stand upon the *Picket*, which is to have one Hand ty'd up as high as it

can

can ſtretch, as he ſtands upon his Toe of one Foot, upon a little Stake drove into the Ground for that Purpoſe, ſo that they neither ſtand nor hang, nor can they change Feet to eaſe themſelves

Pieces, ſignify Cannon As Battering Pieces, ſuch as are us'd at Sieges, and are generally 24 Pounds Field pieces that carry about 10 or 12 Pound Balls, generally planted in the *Van*, as the heavy Cannon is in the main Battle.

Pike A Weapon for a Foot-Soldier made of a long Staff, ſmall and round, and arm'd at the end with a ſharp Iron Spear Generally in a Company of Foot, the two Thirds are Musketeers, and the others Pikemen The Pikes are 14 or 16 Foot long When a Batalion is form'd to engage Horſe in open Field, the Pikes are ſo order'd, that they may face and charge every way, to cover not only the Musketeers, but the Colours, Drums and Baggage Bayonettes, or ſhort Swords, made to clap into the Muzzles of Muskets, ſerve very well inſtead of Pikes

Pioneers Sometimes Men brought in from the Country to Work, but for the moſt part, the Soldiers perform this Duty

A Place, It is commonly us'd to ſignify the Body of a Fortreſs

Place of Arms Thus abſolutely taken, is a ſtrong City choſen for the chief Magazine of an Army

Plac of Arms in a Garrison. A large pen Spot of Ground, either in the midst the City where the great Streets meet, between the Ramparts and the Houses r the Garrison to Rendezvous in upn any sudden Alarm, or other C n-

Place of Arms of an Attack, or Trench A st near it, shelter'd by a Parapet, or *ulment*, for Horse and Foot to be at r Arms, to make good the Trenches nst the Sallies of the Enemies These s are sometimes cover'd by a *Rideau*, Rising Ground, or else by a *Cavin*, or ep Valley, which saves the trouble of tifying them with Parapets, Fascines, bions Barrels, or Bags of Earth They e always open in the Rear, for their tter Communication with the Camp hen the Trench is carry'd on to the *us*, they make it very wide, that it ay serve for a Place of Arms

Place of Arms of a Camp A spacious ece of Ground at the Head of the Camp, draw out the Army in order of Battle.

Plac of Arms of a Troop of Horse, or *Comy of Foot n the Camp* The Spot of ound on which the Troop or Compa- draws out

Plan, or Ichnography The Draught on e Ground of any Fortification, shewing e length of its Lines, the Angles they rm, the distances between them, the eadth of the Moats, and thickness of e Ramparts and Parapets So that a

Plan

Plan represents a Work as it would appear on the plain Field, were it cut off
level with the Foundation, but it does
not shew the heighth and depth of the
several Parts of the Work, which belongs to the *Profile*, and this does not represent the length, it being common to
them both to express the breadth and
thickness of each Part

Platform Vide *Battery*

Platoon, or rather *Peloton* A small
square Body of Musketeers, such as i
us'd to be drawn out of a Batalion of
Foot, when they form the hollow Squar
to strengthen the Angles The Granadiers are generally thus posted *Peloton* i
the *French* Word, from whom we took i
and the vulgar Corruption has brought i
to be pronounc'd *Platoon*

Point-blank Is the Shot of a Gun le-
vell'd in a direct Line, without mounting or sinking the Muzzle, which is us'
for Battery of Works, and sweeping nea
at hand The Point-blank of any common large Cannon is not above 18
Paces

Polygon The Figure or Spot of Groun
that is to be, or is fortified

Interior Polygon The main Body of th
Work, or Town, excluding the Ou-
works

Exterior Polygon The Out-lines of a
the Works, drawn from one outmo
Angle to another quite about

Regul

Regular Polygon That whose Sides and ngles are equal to one another

Irregular Polygon That which has unequal Sides and Angles

Pont de Jonc Vide *Bridge*

Ponton, or *Floating Bridge* An Invenon to pass over a Water It is made of o great Boats, plac'd at some distance om one another, both plank'd over, as the Interval between them, with Rails the Sides, the whole so strong built, at it can carry over Horse and Canon

Pont Volant Vide *Bridge*

Portcullis, *Herse*, or *Sarrazine* Several eat Pieces of Wood laid a-cross one other, and pointed at the Ends with on, the whole like a Harrow These d use to hang over the Gate-ways of rtify'd Places, to be ready to let drop own into the said Gate-way to keep t an Enemy that should come by Surize, if there should not be Time or pportunity to shut the Gates But e *Orgues* are counted better Vide *gues*

Post Any Spot of Ground, whether rtify'd or not, which is capable of dging Soldiers So we say, To gain Post with Sword in Hand; To relieve e Posts, that is, the Guards of the sts

Advanc'd Post A Spot of Ground bere the other Posts, to secure those bend

Postern A ſmall Door in the Flank of a Baſtion, or other part of a Garriſon, to march in and out unperceiv'd by the Enemy, either to relieve the Works, or to make Sallies

Pouches; Are ſuch as the Granadiers have to carry their Hand-Granades in, being of Leather, with a Spring to open and ſhut, large, and hanging by the Soldiers Side

Powder A Compoſition of Charcoal duſt, Salt-petre and Brimſtone, too well known to require any further Account to be given of it

Preſent, Is to hold the Musket Breaſt high, upon a Level, againſt the Soldier's Breaſt, or Shoulder, ready cock'd, to fire upon an Enemy

Prieſts Cap Vide *Bonet a Preſtre*

Primer, Is a Bandaleer, which carries the Powder for Priming of the Musket or a Horn for Priming of Cannon

To Prime, Is to put Powder into the Pan of ſmall Arms, or on the Touch hole of great Guns

Poiſe To Poiſe the Musket, is to hold it in the Right Hand under the Lock, with the Muzzle upright, clear from the Body

Proclamation Vide *Ban*

Profile Vide *Orthographical Section*

Proviſions Are all ſorts of Food for the Army

Provoſt Marſhal An Officer appointed to ſeize and ſecure Deſerters, and all

other

other Criminals, and to set Rates on Provisions in the Army. He has a Lieutenant and a Clerk, and a Troop of Provost's or Marshal's Men a Horseback, as also an Executioner.

Push the Pike. The Pike being charg'd, as describ'd before, the Man thrusts it forward with his Right Hand, advancing the Left with it at the same time, and so draws it back to the Posture it was in before, which is to oppose Horse or Foot advancing to break in upon the Batalion.

Q

QUadrant. An Instrument which is the fourth part of a Circle; and therefore call'd by this Name, us'd by Gunners for Levelling, Mounting, or Imbasing their Pieces.

To Quadrat, or Square a Piece. Is to see whether it is duly plac'd, and well pois'd on the Carriage and Wheels.

Quarter, or Quarters, has several Significations in Martial Affairs.

Quarter, Signifies the sparing of Mens Lives, and giving good Treatment to Enemies vanquish'd. So we say, The Conquerors offer'd good Quarter. The Enemy ask'd Quarter. We gave no Quarter.

A Quarter, signifies not only the Ground a Body of Men incamps on, but the Troops themselves. Therefore we say,

ſay, To beat up the Enemies Quarte[rs]
Such a Quarter is well fortify'd

A Quarter at a Siege An Incampme[nt] upon any of the principal Avenues of t[he] Place, either Commanded by the Gene[ral] of the Army, and then call'd the King['s] or the General's Quarter, or by a Lie[u]tenant-General

Winter-Quarters, Sometimes is tak[en] for the Interval of Time between t[wo] Campaigns, but more generally for t[he] Place or Places where Troops are Lodg['d] during the Winter So we ſay, T[he] Army is marching into Winter Qua[rters] The Winter Quarters are ſettled, T[he] Winter Quarters will be but ſhort

Quarters of Refreſhment The Place or P[la]ces. where Troops, that have been mu[ch] haraſs'd, are put in to recover themſelv[es] during ſome time of the Summer, or Seaſ[on] for the Campaign This is often done [in] hot Countries during the violent Hea[t]

Quartermaſter An Officer, whoſe pri[n]cipal Buſineſs is to look after the Qu[ar]ters of the Soldiers There is a Qu[ar]termaſter-General of the Army Eve[ry] Regiment of Foot has a Quarterm[a]ſter, and every Troop of Horſe one

Queue d'yronde, or *Swallow's-Tail* A D[e]tach'd or Out work, whoſe Sides op[en] towards the Head, or Campaign, a[nd] draw cloſer or narrower towards t[he] Gorge There are Single and Dou[ble] *Tenailles*, and *Horn-works*, call'd by t[he] Name of *Queue d'yronde*, or *Swallow's T[ail]*

becaule their Sides, instead of being pa-
llel, open towards the Head, and grow
arrow at the Gorge, as was said before
When these Works are cast up before the
ront of a Place, they have this Fault,
That they do not sufficiently cover the
lanks of the opposite Bastions, but be-
des that, Engineers sometimes must
ork according to the Ground and Si-
uation, they have this Advantage, that
hey are extraordinary well flank'd by
he Place, which discovers all the length
f their Sides the better Vide *Tenaille*

R

A *Rabanet* The smallest Piece of Cannon but one, being one Inch nd four Eights Diameter in the Bore, ve Foot six Inches long, 300 Pounds Weight, takes a Charge of 6 Ounces of owder, and carries a Shot one Inch and hree Eights Diameter, and Eight Ounces Weight The Point-blank shot of the iece is 70 Paces

To Raise a Siege Is to give over the ttack of a Place, and to quit the Works hrown up against it, and the Posts taken bout it

Rammer or *Scourer*, Is a Rod belonging o all Fire-Arms, proportionable to the ength and Bore of them, serving to hrust down the Powder and Ball, and ress them close, that the Shot may come ut with the more Force Pistols and Muskets have them under the Stock, with mall Plates or Rings which hold them

fast

fast. For Cannon, they are carry'd loose with a Spunge to cleanse those Guns that no Fire may remain in them when discharg'd

Rampart Some will call it *Rampire* but improperly The great Massy Bank of Earth rais'd about a Place to resist the Enemies great Shot, and cover the Buildings On it is rais d a Parapet toward the Campaign It is not to be above three Fathom high, and ten or twelve in thickness,unless more Earth be taken out of the Ditch than can be otherwise bestow'd The Rampart of Half-Moons is the better for being low,that the Musket of the Defendants may the better reach the bottom of the Ditch, but it must be such as is not to be commanded by the *Covert way*

Ranforce-ring of a Gun That which is next before the Touch-hole, between it and the *Trunnions*

Rank The strait Line the Soldiers of a Batalion or Squadron make, as they stand Side by Side To double the Ranks is to put two Ranks into one, so the Files are the thinner, and the Ranks the closer fill'd.

Ration A Day's Allowance of Bread or of Forrage, given to every Man and Horse

Ravelin, Is like the Point of a Bastion, with the Flanks cut off, as consisting of only two Faces, which make an *Angle Saillant* It is plac'd before a Curtin, to cove cover the opposite Flanks of the two next Bastions, or to cover a Bridge and Gate, being always beyond the Moat Only Engineers now use this word *Ravelin*, for the Soldiers generally call it *a Half Moon* Vide *Half-Moon*

Razant Line of Defence *Razant* Vide *Line*

Rear, in general, is the hindmost part of the Army, or the Ground behind it

Rear, or *Rear-Guard* The last of the three Lines of an Army drawn up in *Batalia*, whereof the first is the *Van* or *Van-Guard*, the second the *Main Body*, and the last the *Rear-Guard*, or, by another Name, the *Corps de Reserve*, or *Body of Reserve*. Vide *Line*

Rear-Rank The last Rank of a Batalion, or Squadron

Rear Half-Files The three hindmost Ranks, when a Batalion is drawn up six deep

Recoil of Cannon The Motion, or Run, it takes backward when fir'd, caus'd by the force of the Fire, which when the Piece is discharg'd, seeking every way to fly out, drives the Gun back, and the Powder and Ball forwards A Cannon generally recoils ten or twelve foot, to lessen which, the Platform of the Batteries is commonly made to incline or stoop a little towards the *Embrasures*

Recruits New Men rais'd to strengthen the Forces on foot, either to make the Troops

Troops and Companies more numerou[s] than they were at first, or to fill up th[e] Places of Men kill'd

Rectangle Vide *Triangle*.

Redans or *Indented Works*; Are Line[s] that form several Angles, in and out, t[o] flank one another The Parapet of th[e] *Covert-way* is for the most part carry'd o[n] after this manner, and the same is don[e] on the Sides of a Place that are next to [a] Marsh, or River Vide *Indented Line*

Redoute A small Square Fort, to ser[ve] for a *Corps de Garde* They are us'd t[o] secure the Lines of Circumvallation an[d] Contravallation, and the Approache[s] They are also made sometimes upon ever[y] Traverse of the Trenches to defend th[e] Workmen against the Sallies of the Be[-] sieg'd They are often us'd before stron[g] Towns, at small Distances before th[e] Counterscarp, to keep the Enemy at [a] Distance, and cover the Sallies of th[e] Garrison These *Redoubts* are sometime[s] greater, and sometimes less, but thei[r] Parapet not being to resist Cannon, is on[-] ly 8 or 9 Foot thick, with two or thre[e] Foot-banks, and the Ditch about the sam[e] breadth and depth

Reform To Reform, is to reduce [a] Body of Men, either disbanding th[e] whole, and putting the Officers and M[en] into other Bodies, or only breaking a par[t] and retaining the rest

Reform'd Officer He whose Company o[r] Troop is broke or disbanded, and yet h[e]

con

ntinu'd in Whole or Half Pay, still
serving his Right of Seniority, and
ntinuing in the Way of Preferment

Regiment A Body of several Troops
Horse, or Companies of Foot, and
mmanded by a Colonel Independent
mpanies belong to no Regiment The
mber of Troops or Companies that are
form a Regiment has never been ascer-
n'd, no more than the number of Men
are to form a Troop or Company
there are Regiments of Horse of
Men, and some in *Germany* of 2000
there are Regiments of Foot of 12 or
Companies, which may make 7 or
Men, and the Regiment of *Picardy*
France consists of 120 Companies,
ich at Fifty in a Company amount to
oo Men

Regiments of Guards Vide *Guards*

Regular Attacks Vide *Attacks*

Relais Vide *Foreland*

Relieve To Relieve the Guard, or
lieve the Trenches, is to bring fresh
en upon the Guard, or into the Tren-
es, and send those to Rest that have been
ing Duty there before

Remount To Remount the Cavalry, is
furnish Horses for those who have had
eirs kill'd, or disabled

Rendezvous The Place where Troops
e to assemble.

Reserve, or *Corps de Reserve.* Vide *Line*
Battle, and *Rear-Guard*

Reti-

Retirade A Retrenchment, commo ly consisting of two Faces, which m an Angle inwards, and rais'd in the Bo of a Work that is intended to be l Foot by Foot, when the first Defen are broke down Sometimes it is a Tren with a Parapet, and sometimes it is on made of Fascines loaded with Earth, Gabions, of Barrels or Bags full of Ear with a Ditch, or without, and with P lisades, or without

Retraite Vide *Foreland*

Retrenchment; Is taken for any sort Work, or Intrenchment, or Defen with a Ditch and Brest-work, but m properly it is that which is behind an ther, as when Men are beaten from o Post, they throw up another Retrenc ment within it Sometimes Retrenc ments are call'd *Cutting, off*, and inde both Words signifie the same thing, o ly the first is *French* The Name is prop because that Part of the Defence, whi was lost, is cut off by the new Wo Vide *Intrenchments*

Returns of the Mine. Vide *Gal'ry*

Returns of the Trench The several Ben ings and Oblique Lines of the Trench drawn in some measure parallel to t Sides of the Place attack'd, to prevent b ing enfiladed, or having the Enemi Shot scour along the Length of the Lin These Returns make a great Distance b tween the Tail and the Head of the Tre ches, which are but at a small Distan

t

he straight way Therefore when the Head is attack'd by any Sally, the Vo-unteers and Braves among the Besiegers eap over the Line, and run out of all helter to repulse the Sally, and cut off he Enemies Retreat

Rev rse, signifies on the Back, or be-ind So we say, a Reverse View, a Re-erse Commanding Ground, a Reverse attery

Review. The Appearance of any Body f Troops under Arms, to be view'd hether they are compleat as to Num-ers, and well condition'd

Rhine-land Rod A Measure us'd in Fo-fication by *Dutch* Engineers, being two athom, or twelve Foot.

Rhomboid A Figure that has the op-osite Sides and Angles equal, yet neither l the Sides, nor all the Angles, but on- two of each

Rhombus, or *Lozange.* A Square Figure hat has the four Sides equal, but not he Angles, whereof two are obtuse, and wo acute It is what we vulgarly call *amant-cut*, like the Glass of old Win-ows.

Rideau A small rising Ground run-ing along a Plain, and sometimes almost arallel to the Front of a Place, to which is very prejudicial, as being a Work eady thrown up to cover the Enemy is properly so call'd, because *Rideau* in *rench* is a Curtin, and this is, as it were, a Curtin drawn by Nature to hide Men from the Town

Round A Watch commanded by an Officer that goes in the Night about the Ramparts of a ſtrong Place, to obſerve whether the Sentinels are watchful upon their Duty, or in the Streets of a Town, to keep good order

To Roul Officers of equal Quality, who mount the ſame Guards, and do the ſame Duty, relieving one another, are ſaid to Roul, as Captains with Captains, and Subalterns with Subalterns They command one another according to the Date of their Commiſſions

To Run the Gauntlet When a Soldier has committed ſome conſiderable Offence, and is ſentenc'd to run the Gauntlet, the Regiment is drawn up making a Lane with every Man a Wand in his Hand, the Criminal runs through with his Back naked, and every Man has a Stroke at him If it be intended to make the Puniſhment rigorous, the Officers have a watchful Eye to ſee that the Men do not favour the Criminal, and puniſh any that preſumes ſo to do.

S.

S*Ac-a-Terre* Vide *Canvas Bags*

Safe-Guard A Protection the Prince or his General gives to ſome of the Enemies Country to be ſecur'd from being ravag'd by his Men, or quartering them

Sol

Soldiers left in ſuch Places to ſecure them againſt their own Men, are call'd *Safe-Guards*

Saker, the loweſt Sort A Cannon three Inches and four Eights Diameter in the Bore, eight Foot long, 1400 Pounds Weight Its Charge of Powder three Pounds ſix Ounces, and carries a Bullet three Inches and two Eights Diameter, and four Pounds twelve Ounces Weight. The Point-blank Shot of it 150 Paces.

Saker Ordinary. A Gun three Inches ſix Eights Diameter in the Bore, nine Foot long, 1500 Pounds Weight, takes four Pounds for its Charge of Powder, and carries a Bullet three Inches and four Eights Diameter, and ſix Pounds Weight. Its Point-blank Shot 160 Paces

Saker of the largeſt Size Four Inches Diameter in the Bore, ten Foot long, 1800 Pounds Weight Its Charge 5 Pounds of Powder, the Diameter of its Shot three Inches and 6 Eights, the Weight of it ſeven Pounds five Ounces, the Point-blank Shot of the Piece 163 Paces

A Sally In French, *Sortie* The iſſuing out of the Beſieg'd from their Works, and falling upon the Beſiegers to cut them off, and deſtroy their Works, as they often do in ſucceſsful Sallies, killing many Men, deſtroying the Trenches and Batteries, and nailing the Cannon. To make a Sally, to repulſe a Sally; to cut off a Sally, that is, to get between them that made it and Home.

Salute A Discharge of Cannon or Small-shot, or both, in Honour of some Person of extraordinary Quality The Colours also salute Royal Persons and Generals, which is done bowing them down to the Ground

Sappe A deep Trench carry'd far into the Ground, and descending by Steps from top to bottom, so that it covers on the Side, and to cover over Head they lay a-cross it *Madriers*, that is, thick Planks or Clays, that is, Branches of Trees close bound together, and throw Earth over them to secure them against Fire Formerly, this Word *Sappe* signified a Hole dug under a Building, in order to overthrow it When a *Covert-way* is well defended by Musketeers, the Besiegers must make their way down into it by *Sappe* Vide *Descent*

Sarrazine Vide *Portcullisses*

Saucisse A long Train of Powder roll'd up in a Pitch-Cloth, and sew'd together in length, so that it reach from the *Fourneau*, or Chamber of the Mine, to the Place where the Engineer stands to spring the Mine It may be about two Inches Diameter There are generally two *Saucisses* to every Mine, that if the one fails the other may hit

Saucissons, or *Saucisses* Faggots made of the Bodies of Underwood, or of the large Branches of great Trees, wherein they differ from Fascines, which are of small Wood. The *Saucisson* is bound in the Middl dle and at both Ends, and serves to cover the Men, make Epaulments, and for other Uses.

Scalade, or *Escalade* A furious Attack upon a Wall or Rampart, carry'd on with Ladders to mount, without going on in form, or carrying on Works to secure the Men

A Scale A Rule us'd by Engineers to draw Fortifications on Paper, and another sort us'd by Gunners to take the Dimensions of their Guns

Scalene Vide *Triangle*

Scarp The inward Slope of the Ditch of a Place, that is, the Slope of that Side of the Ditch which is next to the Place, and faces towards the Campaign

Scenography The Prospect of a fortify'd Place, as it appears to the Eye, when from without we look upon any Side of it, and observe its Situation, Enclosure, Steeples, and Tops of the Houses

To Scour the length of a Line. To rake it from End to End with the Shot; so that every Bullet which comes in at one End, sweeps all along to the other, and leaves no Place of Security in it

Scourer Vide *Rammer*

Second Captain, or *Lieutenant en Second*. One whose Company has been broke, and he is joyn'd to another, to act and serve under the Captain or Lieutenant of it, and receive Pay as Reform'd There are also Second Captains, and Lieutenants of the first Creation, that is, who were never so in the other Companies; but particularly, Second Lieute-nants are much us'd among the Foot in *France*

Seniority The Order of Time elaps'd since the first raising of a Regiment, or an Officer's receiving his Commission. In the Line of Battle, the Squadrons of Horse are posted on the Right or Left of the Line, according to the Seniority of the Officers, that is, of their Commissions; for the Colonels of Horse command by the Seniority of their Commissions, but this Method is not observ'd among the Foot, for their Colonels have Precedence and Command according to the Seniority of their Regiments The Captains in the same Regiment of Horse or Foot, roul, and have place among themselves, according to the Seniority of Commission, and their Troops or Companies have no Preference one before the other, but by the Dates of their Captains Commissions. The first Captain failing, his Company, of the first, becomes the last of the Batalion, and the second becomes the first. As for Subalterns, the Seniority of their Commissions does not alter their Post but they roul, and ascend or descend with their Companies

Sentinel A private Soldier taken out of the *Corps de Garde* and posted upon any Spot of Ground, to stand and watch carefully for the Security of the said Guard of any Body of Troops or Post, and prevent any Surprize from the Enemy

Ser

Sentinel Perdue A Sentinel posted near an Enemy in some very dangerous Post, where he is in hazard of being lost

Serjeant An Officer without Commission in a Company of Foot, or Troop of Dragoons Sometimes he commands small Detachments, and among other Things, it is his particular Duty to see the Men keep their due Distances, and to straiten the Ranks and Files, to receive and carry Orders between the Major and his Officers, and the Company, and go the *Patrouills, &c* Generally common Companies have two Serjeants each He must read and write, and his Weapon is a Halbard

Serjeant-Major Vide *Major*

Shot All sorts of Bullets for whatsoever Fire Arms, from the Cannon to the Pistol Those for Cannon are of Iron, those for Musket, Carabine, and Pistol, of Lead At Sea, they use Chain and Bar-shot, which are two half Bullets joyn'd by an Iron Bar or Chain, which gives them Length to cut all they meet with Vide *Bullet*

Shovels Us'd in all Works too well known, and need no Description

Shoulder of a Bastion Vide *Epaul*

Shoulder your Arms, Is to lay the Musket on the left Shoulder, holding it with the left Hand on the Hollow between the But-end and the Lock The Pike is laid upon the right Shoulder, holding it with the right Hand, so that the

the But-end may come within a Foot of the Ground, sloping so, that, the Spear may be reasonably mounted behind

Sides of Hornworks, Crown-works, Tenailles, and such-like Outworks, by the *French* call'd *Ailes*, or *Wings*, are the Ramparts and Parapets that enclose them on the Right and Left from the Gorge to the Head These Sides, when they are not longer than Musket-shot, are generally strait Lines, because then they are flank'd from the Place But if the Sides are above Musket shot, they are sometimes indented, or made with *Redans*, or else there are Traverses, or cross Intrenchments, cut in their Ditch So that it is more dangerous attacking the Sides of these Works, than the Head.

Siege. The incamping of an Army about a Place it designs to attack, the whole Time it lies before it, and all it does for reducing of it So we say, to lay Siege, to carry on a Siege, To raise a Siege.

Sillon A Work rais'd in the midst of a Ditch to defend it, when it is too wide This Work, as it runs, forms little Bastions, Half-Moons, or Redans, or Indentures, which are lower than the Rampart of the Place, but higher than the *Covert-way* This Name of *Sillon* is going out of use, and they now call it *Envelope* Vide *Envelope*, *Counter Guard* and *Lunette*

Single Tenaille Vide *Tenaille*.

Sixain, An ancient Order of Battle for six Batalions, which, supposing them to be all in a Line, is form'd thus. The Second and Fifth Batalions advance and constitute the Van, the First and Sixth fall back into the Rear, or *Corps de Reserve*, and the Third and Fourth, remain on the same Ground for the Main Battle. Every Batalion ought to have a Squadron of Horse on its Right, and another on its Left. Any Number of Batalions produc'd by the Multiplication of six, may be drawn up in this Order, for twelve Batalions will make two *Sixains*, eighteen will make three, and so on. Vide *Cinquain*.

Skirmish, A small Encounter of a few Men when they fight in Confusion without observing Order.

Slings, Are Leather Thongs, made fast to both ends of the Musket, and serving for the Men to hang them by on their Shoulders, that so they may have both their Hands free, without laying aside their Fire-Arms.

A Soldier, Is he that is listed, and receives Pay, to serve his Prince or State in the Wars, either a Foot or a Horseback.

To Sound the Trumpet. Vide *Trumpet*.

Spades, for throwing up Works, do not need any more should be said of them.

Sponge, A long Staff with a Roul at one end, cover'd with a Sheep-skin of the bigness of the Bore of a Gun, to scour it after firing, that no Fire may remain within.

 Spurs

Spurs Are Walls that cross a part of the Rampart, and join to the Town Wall

Squadron A Body of Horse, the number not fix'd, but from an hundred to two hundred Men, sometimes more and sometimes less, according as Generals think fit, the Army is in strength, and occasion requires

Square A Figure compos'd of four equal Sides, and four Right Angles

Long Square, Has Right Angles but two of the Sides are long, and the other two short

A Square Body, Which has as many Men in File, as in Rank, and is equal whatsoever way it faces

Hollow Square A Body of Foot drawn up with an empty Space in the middle for the Colours, Drums and Baggage, facing and cover'd by the Pikes every way, to oppose the Horse

Staff Officer Vide *Officer*

Star-Redoute, of four, of five, of six or of more Points, otherwise call'd an *Estoile* These are all small Forts, or Redoubts, with Angles Saillant, and returning or entring These are not much in use now, because their Angle inwards is not Flank'd, and the Square Redoubts are sooner built, and as serviceable

Stock of a Gun, or Pistol, is the wooden Part, unto which the Barril is fix'd, for the conveniency of Handling and Firing

Straw. For Straw is a Word of Command, to dismiss the Soldiers when they have grounded their Arms, so that they be ready to return to them upon the first Firing of a Musket, or Beat of Drum

Subaltern Vide *Officer*

Sub-Brigadier, *Sub-Lieutenant*, and the like, are Under-Officers appointed for the ease of those over them of the same Denomination Sub-Lieutenants of Foot take their Post at the Head of the Pikes

Subsistance Is Money paid Weekly, or Monthly or otherwise, to Soldiers, for them to subsist on till the general Pay-days, when their Accounts are made, and then receive what more is due to them, for the Subsistance is always less than the Pay

Sub-Divisions, Are the lesser Parcels, into which a Regiment is divided in Marching, being half the greater Divisions

Succour To Succour a Place is to raise the Siege, driving the Enemy from before it

Superficial Fourneau Vide *Caisson*

Surface Is that part of the Exterior Side, which is terminated by the Flank, prolong'd or extended and the Angle of the nearest Bastion The double of this Line with the Curtin, is equal to the Exterior Side

Sutler, Is one that follows the Camp, and sells all sorts of Provisions to the Sol-

Soldiers. In all Garrisons there are also Sutlers, who serve the Soldiery

Swallow's-Tail Vide *Queue d'yronde*

T

TAil of the Trenches The first Work the Besiegers make, when they open the Trenches, as the Head of the Attack is carry'd on towards the Place There is always Danger at the Tail of the Trenches, because it is exposed to the Batteries of the Place and the Cannon, mounted on the Cavalier, plays upon those that Relieve and Mount the Guard, A Guard of Horse is ever kept at the Tail of the Trenches, to be in a readiness to come to the Relief of Workmen at the Head, in case of Sallies, and this Guard is reliev'd as often as the Trenches.

Talus. The Slope allow'd to every Work rais'd of Earth, that it may stand the faster, and is more or less, according as the Earth is looser or more binding As for Instance, the Rampart is not built upright, because it is of Earth, but it goes sloping, being thicker at the bottom or foot, than at the top, and this Slope is call'd the *Talus*

Inward Talus The Slope of the Rampart, or other Work next the Place, which is commonly double the outward *Talus* of that same Work.

Outward Talus The Slope allow'd the Work on the outside from the Place, and towards the Campaign

Tato Sometimes call'd, The Retreat, the Beat of Drum at Night for all Soldiers in Garrison to repair to their Quarters, and to their Tents in the Field After which, in Frontier Towns, and where the Inhabitants are suspected, they are not permitted to stir abroad, or at least not without a Light

Te Deum A Holy Hymn sung in Thanksgiving for any Victory obtain'd; which is often abus'd, being sung by those that are beaten to conceal their Shame

Temoins Vide *Witnesses*

Tenaille Has several Significations in Fortification, as,

Tenaille of a Place, or *Fortress* The Faces of it Vide *Face*

Tenaille An Outwork, whereof there are two Sorts, the Single, and the Double

The Single Tenaille A Work, the Head whereof is form'd by two Faces, making one Angle Rentrant, or Inwards, and whose Sides run directly Parallel from the Head to the Gorge

The Double Tenaille A Work whose Head is form'd by four Sides, which make two Angles Rentrant, or Inwards, and three Angles Saillant, and whose Sides run strait from the Head to the Gorge. When these Sides are Parallel, the Single or Double *Tenailles* are known by no other Name, but when there is more breadth at the Head, than at the Gorge, they are call'd *Queue d'yronde*, or Swallows-Tails. *Tenailles* are faulty in this respect, That they are not flank'd or defended towards their Dead, or Inward Angle, because the heighth of the Parapet hinders seeing down before that Angle, so that the Enemy can lodge himself there under Covert. Therefore *Tenailles* are only made when there is not time enough to make a Horn-work.

Terre-plain. The Superficies of the Rampart, being the plain Space or Way on it, Parallel to the level of the Ground, and bounded next the Campaign by the Parapet, and next the Place by the Interior *Talus*.

Tent. The *Tents* are of a close Cloth, or Canvas for the Soldiers to lye in, when in the Field. Four or five Soldiers lye in one small Tent, the Officers have greater, according to their several Posts. They are always pitcht regularly, every Regiment apart, and each Troop or Company in a Line, or File, the Officers in the Rear, the whole composing orderly Streets.

To Tertiate a Piece. Is to try a Cannon, whether it has its due thickness of Metal in all Parts.

Toise. A Fathom, or Six Foot.

Tong. The same as *Tenaille*.

Touch-hole, is a small Hole in all Fire-Arms passing through the Barril to the Chamber where the Charge lyes for the Powder on the outside to convey the Fire to that within

Town-Major Vide *Major*

Trail the Pike, is to hold the Spear-end in the Right Hand, about a Hand's breadth from the Spear, the flat of the Spear lying upwards, the But end on the Ground behind the Man

Trapeze A Figure that has only two of its four Sides parallel

Trapezoide, or *Tablet* Has all its four Sides and Angles unequal, and no Sides Parallel

Traverse A Trench with a Parapet, and sometimes two, one on the Right, and another on the Left Sometimes this Trench is open over Head, and sometimes cover'd with Planks loaded with Earth This Word is often taken for a Gallery, and also signifies a Retrenchment, or Line fortify'd with Fascines, Barrils, or Bags of Earth, or Gabions

Trench In general it signifies any Ditch, or Cut made in the Earth

Trenches, *Approaches* or *Attacks* Are Works carry'd on by the Besiegers, being cut into the Ground with Parapets for their Men to gain Ground, and draw near the Fortifications of the Place under Covert They are carry'd on differently, according to the nature of the

 Ground.

Ground For if, all round the Town the Ground be Rocky, the Trenches are rais'd above it with Fascine, or Faggots Baggs of Earth, Gabions, Wool-packs, Epaulments of Earth brought from a far, and any Thing that may cover the Men without flying, as Stones, and the like But, if the Earth is fit to dig, the Trenches are no other than a Ditch, or Way sunk down into the Earth, and edg'd with a Parapet next the Besieged Its Depth is about six or seven Foot and its Breadth seven or eight How soever the Trenches be made, they must always be so contriv'd, that the Besieg'd may never Enfilade them, that is, Scour the length of them with their Shot For this Reason they are carried on by Coudes or Traverses, which are Lines returning back from the End of them and running almost Parallel with the Place

To open Trenches To begin to dig, or work upon the Line of Approaches, which is generally done in the Night sometimes within Musket-shot, and sometims within half, or even within whole Cannon-shot of the Place, if there be no Hollows, nor Rising Grounds about it; and the Garrison is strong and their Cannon well serv'd The Workmen that open the Trenches are always supported by Bodies of Men against the Sallies of the Besiegers, and sometimes those Bodies lie between them and nd the Place, and on their Right and Left The Pioneers sometimes work on their Knees, and the Men that are to support them lie flat on their Faces, both to avoid the Shot from the Place The Pioneers are generally cover'd with Mantlets, or Saucissons

To mount the Trenches. To go upon Duty into the Trenches

To Relieve the Trenches To Relieve those that are upon Duty in them

To carry on the Trenches To advance them towards the Place

Triangle, or Trigon A Figure consisting of Three Sides, and as many Angles

Triangle Rectangle. Which has one Right Angle

Triangle Ambligone Which has an Obtuse Angle

Triangle Oxigon. Which has three sharp, or acute Angles

Triangle Equilateral Which has all three Sides of an equal Length

Triangle Isosele. Which has only two Sides equal

Triangle Scalene. Which has all three Sides unequal

Trigger, Is a small piece of Iron plac'd under the Lock of any Fire-Arms, drawing which back, when the Piece is cock'd, the Cock falls, and giving Fire to the Powder in the Pan, the Shot goes off

Trigon. Vide *Triangle.*

A Troop A small Body of Horse, o Dragoons, the number not determin'd but usually about 50, under the Com mand of a Captain

Independent Troop. That which is no incorporated in any Regiment

Troop To beat the Troop, Is the se cond Beat of Drum when the Foot are march, the General being the first give notice of the March, and the Troo the next for the Men to repair to the Colours.

Trooper. The vulgar Name, by whi every Horse-Soldier is call'd. The *Fren* call them *Maitres*, or *Cavaliers*

Trumpet, Signifies either the Marti Instrument us'd among the Horse to gi notice what they are to do, or the M that sounds it To sound to Horse, March, a Charge or Retreat, a L vet Every Troop of Horse has a Trum pet

Trunion-Ring The Ring about a Ca non next before the *Trunion*

Trunions Two Pieces of Metal stick out of the Sides of a Piece, about t middle of it, on which it rests, and mounted or imbass'd,

Turn-pike A Piece of Wood or Sp twelve or fourteen Foot long, six eight Inches Diameter, cut in a Sexang lar Form, every Side of it bor'd full Holes about an Inch Diameter, and f or six Inches from one another, but answering on the Sides to one anoth n the contrary all differently posited hrough these Holes, Pickets, that is, ort Pikes, are run, being about five or x Foot long, pointed with Iron, and stned into the Holes with Nails or Vedges Thus the Points stand out eve- y way, and these Turn-pikes are of great se to stop an Enemy, being plac'd on a reach, or at the Entrance of a Camp, in any Gap Turn-pikes are otherwise ll'd *Chevaux de Frise*

V.

V*AN*, or *Vanguard* The first Line of an Army drawn up in Batalia, hich gives the first Charge upon the nemy, the Second Line is the Main Bo- , and the Third the Rear-Guard, or Bo- y of Reserve The *Van* is the Fron , or remost Part of any Body or Bodies of en

I dette A Sentinel of the Horse

To View a Place. To ride about it be- re forming of the Siege, and observe e Strength and Weakness of its Situa- on and Fortification, in order to attack e we kest Part This Care belongs to e General himself

Vivandier One that follows the Army ith Provisions, to sell to the Soldiers hen they have Occasion · From the ench Word *Vivres*, Provisions

Volunteers Gentlemen, who without ving any certain Post, or Employment, in the Forces under Command, put them-selves upon Warlike Expeditions, and ru into Dangers only to gain Honour an Preferment

Uncap your Cartridges; Is to take off th Top of the Paper, which is folded dow at the End, that so the Powder may fa loose to the Touch-hole to take fir which otherwise the Paper would hin-der. This is commonly tore off wit the Teeth.

Ustensile. The Necessaries due to every Soldier, and to be furnish'd by his Ho where he is quarter'd They are, a Be with Sheets, a Pot, a Glass or Cup drink out of, a Dish, a Place at the Fir and a Candle Sometimes the Inhabitant compound, and allow so much in Mone to be eas'd of it.

W

W*Arrant Officer* Vide *Officer* *Way of the Rounds* Vide *Chem des Rondes*, or *Fausse-Braye*.

Well A Depth the Miner sinks in the Ground, and thence carries on t Branches, or Galeries, to find out, an disappoint the Enemies Mines, or to pr pare one

To Wheel This is a Motion that brin a Batalion or Squadion to front on th Side where the Flank was, which Wheeling to the Right or Left, it Enemy appear ready to attack the Fla r, if it be thought fit, to fall upon the nemies Flank In this Motion, the anks and Files must take great Care ot to bend, but every one to keep his ue Distance, and there must be very able erjeants at the Angles, to see the Files o not break and fall into Confusion the Batalion wheels to the Right, the eft Wing moves first, describing the urth Part of a Circle about the File-lea-er on the Right, who is the Center of e Motion, and stirs not off his round If the Wheeling be to the eft, the contrary is perform'd Squa-ons of Horse wheel after the same man-r.

Wing of an Army drawn up for Battle, *Wing* of one of its Lines; Is the orse on the Flanks, or at the End of h Line on the Right and Left

Wing of a Batalion or Squadron. The ght and Left-hand Files that make up h Side or Flank When a Batalion awn up, the Pikes are in the Center, the Musketeers on the Wings, which ngs are also call'd *Great Divisions*, *Whole Divisions* of the Batalion. In heelings, when they wheel to the ght, the Left-wing of the Batalion ves first, whilst the Right Wing takes hort Compass, turning upon the File-der of the first File, as upon a Center. he contrary is done if they wheel to e Left.

Winter Quarters Vide *Quarters*

Witnesses, or *Temoins*, Are certain Parcels of Earth left in the Foundation of those Places that are dug down, in order to make a judgment by them, of how many Cubical Feet, or Fathom of Earth have been dug out

The Word; Is a Word that serves for a Token, and Mark of Distinction, given every Night in an Army by the General, and in Garrison by the Governour, or other Officer commanding in Chief, to prevent Surprize, and hinder an Enemy, or any treacherous Person to pass backwards and forwards When the Governor, Deputy-Governor, or Town-Major go the Rounds in a Garrison, the Officer commanding in every *Corps de Garde*, is to receive and give them the *Word*, but Inferior Rounds are to give the Word to the Guard

Word of Command Vide *Command*

Works; Are all the Fortifications about any Place, as Out-works are those without the first Enclosure

Y

YOunger Regiment or Officer That Regiment is youngeſt which was rais'd, and that Officer youngeſt, whose Commiſſion is of the lateſt Date, tho' he be never ſo old a Man, or have ſerv'd never ſo long in other Capacities; and according to theſe Rules, Regiments and Officers are poſted, and command. See more of it under the Word *Seniority*.

A SEA-

A

SEA-DICTIONARY.

Explaining the SEA-TERMS, the NAMES of each Part of a Ship, its Rigging, and all other Things belonging to it.

A.

ABaft Vide *Aft*

Aft, or *Abaft* In the Sea-Terms signifies Backwards, or Behind, to distinguish what is one or plac'd from the Stem towards the ern of the Ship, as *Come aft*, or *go aft*; at is, come or go backwards, or towards e Stern. *Hale the Sheat aft*, that is, ale back towards the Stern. *A Shot l'd the Ship fore and aft*; that is, it came before, and went out a-Stern. *Abaft e Fore-mast*, backwards from the Fore-ast By which it appears, that the Vord is applicable to any Part of the ip, in respect of those that are towards e Stern.

Aloof, is us'd in conding the Ship when ſhe goes upon a Tack, and is ſpoken from the Conder to the Steers-man when he ſuffers the Ship to fall off from the Wind, and does not keep her ſo near by a Wind as ſhe may well lie

Amain In the common Significa tion is all at once, that is, when they are letting down any thing with th Tackle, which is done letting it deſcen gently, at laſt they cry *Amain*, which i for all the Men who hold the Tackle t let go their Hold at once In this Senſ it is us'd by all Ships; but Men of Wa have a peculiar Application, which i when they encounter another Ship, an cry to them in her, *Amain*, that is, t bid them yield They alſo uſe, *Wavin Amain*, which is waving a Sword, or othe bright Thing, for a Signal to other Shi to ſtrike their Top-ſails Hence, *to ſtri Amain*, is to let fall the Top-ſails at the full run, not gently

Anchor Moſt Men know, the Uſe o an Anchor is to keep a Ship in one Plac and that it conſiſts of a long Iron Shaf at one End whereof are, as it were, Tw Arms in a circular Form, with broad an pointed Flooks at the Ends of them, an at the other End of the ſaid Shaft a Pie of Timber faſten'd the contrary way the Iron Arms The Anchor has the ſeveral Parts, the *Ring*, by which the C ble is made faſt to it; the *Eye*, throu which the Ring paſſes; the *Head*,

wh

which the Eye is; the *Nut*, which holds the Beam, the *Beam*, being Two Pieces of Timber join'd together on the End of the Shank, crossing opposite to the Flooks that they may not lie flat but take hold; the *Shank*, is the long Iron which has the Beam on the one End, and the Flooks at the other, the *Arms*, are the Irons which have the Flooks at their Ends; and the *Flooks* are the Two broad and pointed Ends of the Arms, which take hold in the Ground, and keep the Ship from being carried away by the Wind or Water. The Proportion of Anchors is according to the Bulk of the Ship, which commonly has several Degrees of Anchors, and each of them its peculiar Name, as first, the *Kedge*, or *Kedger*, which is the smallest us'd in kedging down a River Next, a *Stream-Anchor*, us'd in deep Waters to stop a Tide withal in fair Weather The others are call'd the First, Second, and Third Anchors being such as a Ship may ride by in reasonable Weather, and are something bigger one than another When in any Straits or near a Port, they carry Two of these at the Bow, whence they are also call'd the First, Second, and Third Bows The biggest Anchor of all is the *Sheat-Anchor*, frequently by Seamen call'd *Their last Hope*, being us'd in the greatest Extremity, as their last Refuge. The Proportion of these Anchors is according to the Size of the Vessel, for that which would be but a *Kedger* to one

Ship, would be a *Sheat-Anchor* to a smal-ler A Ship of 500 Tun has 2000 Weight allow'd to its *Sheat-Anchor*, and the big-gest Ship has an Anchor of 3500 Weight There are several Terms belonging to the Anchor, as,

The Anchor is a peek, that is, when heaving of it up, the Cable is right per-pendicular betwixt the Haws and the An-chor

The Anchor is a Cock-bell, when the An-chor hangs up and down by the Ship Side, which is when the Ship is ready to come to an Anchor

Let fall the Anchor, is, let it drop down into the Sea

The Anchor is foul, when the Cable by the turning of the Ship, is got about the Flook that is out of the Ground, which will cut the Cable asunder, and make the Anchor not hold, for which Reason when the Ship comes to an Anchor where there is a Tide, they lay out Two Anchors, that the Ship, upon the turning of the Tide, may wind up clear of them both

Clear the Anchor, is, get the Cable off the Flook This Term is also generally us'd when they let fall the Anchor, to see that the Buoy-Rope nor any other hang about it

Fetch or bring home the Anchor, that is, weigh it in the Boat, and bring it aboard the Ship

The Anchor comes home, is when the Ship

d r

rives away with the Tide or Sea, and he Anchor drags after; which may hap en, either if the Anchor be too small or the Ship, or the Ground soft and wzie, in which Places they sometimes hooe the Anchor See *Shooe*

Boat the Anchor, is, put it into the Boat.

Anchorage, or *Anchoring*, is, letting fall he Anchor, or Anchors, into the Sea, ith Cables to them, for the Ship to de fast by them It is also the Place here the Anchor falls, for they say, ere is good Anchoring where there is hole Water, because in deep Waters the ea has more Force against the Ship, and e Anchors are long a weighing. That also good Anchoring where the Ground not too soft or owzie, in which the nchors have no hold, nor yet too hard stony, that may cut the Cables; the st Ground to ride in being a stiff Clay hard Sand, as also where they may de out of the Way of the Tide And stly, where they are Land-lock'd, so as at the Sea-gate can have no Power over em Add to this, If the Lee-Shore on very side be so soft, that if a Ship come ground, she can take no Hurt, or else at she may have Sea-room to set Sail, the Cable breaks, or the Anchor comes ome Any Place that has these Quali- es, is said to afford good *Anchoring*, or *nchorage*, and it is bad Anchoring here they are wanting

Anchor Stock A long Piece of Timbe fitted to and fasten'd at the Nuts of th Anchor, crossing the Flooks, that it ma so guide the Anchor on the Ground that one of the Flooks may be sure t take hold and fasten in the Ground without which the Anchor would lie fla and consequently have no hold It usually proportion'd by the Length o the Shank

Arm of the Anchor, is that Part to whic the Flook is set

To arm a Shot, is to bind some Oakham Rope-Yarn, or old Clouts, about one En of a Cross-Bar Shot, or the like, that th End which goes first out of the Piec may not take hold in any Flaws of which would endanger the breaking o the Gun The same is us'd to lon Pieces of broken Iron, fir'd out of Or nance when they come to boarding, an in small Shot for Muskets

Armed A Ship is said to be well Arm when she is well provided with all Ne cessaries for Fight

Awning, is a Sail, or large Piece o Canvas, or the like, spread over an Part of, or over all, the Ship above th Deck, to keep the Sun off, that the M may take the Air, without being expos to the scorching Heat in the Day, or co Dews in the Night, and is of great U in hot Countries

Ashlace The same is in a Coach o Cart as supporting the Cheeks of the C riages whereon the Piece lies

An

Axletree of the Pump, is the Iron which goes through the Wheel of the Chain-Pump, and bears the Weight of it.

B

BAck-Stayes. Vide *Stayes*.

To Bale, is to lade Water out of the Ship's Hould, with Buckets, Cans, or the like, which is never done but in Extremity, when either the Pumps fail, or the Leak is greater than they can deliver. The former often happens in extraordinary Pumping, when they either draw Wind, or are stoak'd, or some Part of them gives way. Else *Baling* is never us'd, because it delivers little, and tires the Men more.

Bales, are Hoops, the Ends whereof being stuck into the Sides of a Barge, in Mortices made for that purpose, they form an Arch over that Part where the Seats are, and over them is laid the Tilt, to keep off the Sun.

Ballast, is Gravel, Stones, Lead, or any other heavy Goods, laid next the Keelson of the Ship to keep her stiff in the Sea. The best Ballast is the heaviest, and that lies closest, fastest and driest; not only for the Ship's bearing Sail, but for stowing of Goods, the Health of the Crew, and saving of Cask, and other Goods. If a Ship have too much Ballast she will draw too much Water, if too little, she will bear no Sail.

To Trench the Ballast; is to divide it in the Hould, to find a Leak in the Bottom of her.

The Ballast shoots: That is, runs over from one Side to the other, for which Reason all kind of Grain is dangerous Lading, as being apt to shoot, but that they make Bulk-heads of Boards, to keep it from shifting from Side to Side, as the Ship heels upon a Tack.

Bar. Vide *Capstain-Bar*.

A Bar of a Harbour, is a Rock, Sand, or Shelf, lying a-cross the Mouth or Entrance into the Harbour, which cannot be sail'd over but upon the Flood, and generally requires Pilots of the Place to bring Ships in safe.

Bar of the Port, is a Billet, or Piece of Wood thrust through the Shackles to shut fast the Ports.

Barge; is a large handsome Boat belonging to a Ship, much like the Barges we see on Rivers, to carry Captains or other Persons of Note aboard or ashore.

Beak, or *Beak-head*, is that Part which is fasten'd to the Stern of the Ship, and supported with a Knee, fasten'd into the Stern, and call'd the *Main-Knee*, to which is made fast the Coller of the *Main-Stay*. The Fore-Tacks are brought aboard in the *Beak-head*, and there is the Stand, where Men handle most of the Spritsail and Spritsail-Topsail Rigging. It also serves for Ornament to grace the Ship.

The Beak head sleeves, or stands sleeving, that

that is, the outermost End of it stands very much up towards the Boltsprit.

Beam The Beams are those great Cross-Timbers which keep the Sides asunder, and support the Decks, or Orlops, according to whose Strength the Ship is more or less able to carry Ordnance All great and strong Ships have a Tire, or Row of Beams in Hould, on which the Deck lies The *Main-Beam* is ever the next to the *Main-Mast*, at which Place the Breadth of the Ship is measur'd, and from this, the other Beams, both forward and aftward, are call'd the First, Second Third, *&c* beginning at this, which is also call'd *Midship-Beam*

The Beam of the Anchor, is the Piece of Timber fasten'd to the Nuts of the Shank, and standing cross to the Flooks, to keep them from lying flat on the Ground, but that one of them may take hold

To bear, is sometimes spoken in the ordinary Sense, as a Ship will bear much Ordnance, that is, carry much *To bear sail well*, denotes that a Ship is stiff sided, and will not couch down on a side with much Sail

To bear out her Ordnance; is that her Guns lie so high, and she will go so upright, that in reasonable fighting Weather she will be able to keep out her low Tire, and not be forc'd to shut in the Ports

One Ship overbears another that is, can carry more Sail than the other in a great Gale of Wind

To bear with the Land, or *with a Harbour*, or *a Ship*, is to sail towards it when the Ship bears to Windward of it.

To bear under the Lee of a Ship, is when the Ship that is to Weather comes under the other Ship's Stern, and so gives her the Wind, which is the greatest Respect that one Ship can pay to another at Sea.

A Piece will bear more Shot, or *not so much*, that is, will endure a greater Charge, or is over-charg'd.

The Piece comes to bear, signifying that now she lies right with the Mark.

Bear in, when a Ship sails before, or with a large Wind into Harbour or Chanel, or sails large towards the Land, then they say, She bears in with the Chanel, Harbour, or Land. But this Way of Speaking is not us'd if she sails close by a Wind.

Bear off. A Ship is said to bear off from the Land, or another Ship, when she would not come near it, but keeps farther off than her Course lies.

Bear off, is also the common Expression for Thrust off, as when any thing has hold of the Side of the Ship, or the like, they say, *Bear off*, that is, Thrust it off, and so in other Cases.

Bear up, us'd in Conding the Ship when they would have her go larger, or more before the Wind, than she did.

Bear up round, is to put her right before the Wind, or to bring her by the Lee, which is done by thrusting the Helm up to Windward, as close as it will go to the Ship's Side

Becalm'd, is when there is no Wind stirring to fill the Sails, so that the Ship has no Way, but lies in the same Place, or only carried by the Stream or Current A Ship is also said to be becalm'd by the Land, when that keeps the Wind from her, and by another Ship, when she comes so close as to hinder her from the Wind

Beds, are a sort of false Decks, rais'd on the Deck of the Ship, when this is too low from the Ports, so that the Carriages cannot mount the Ordnance sufficiently, but that they will lie too near the *Port-wast* or *Gun-Wale*, and these Beds raise them higher, and fit to traverse The Bed is also that Plank in the Carriage of a Gun which lies under the Breech of the Piece on which the Quoins do lie

To Belay; is to make fast any running Rope when it is hal'd as much as is necessary, as the *Hallyards*, when they hoyse a Yard, or the Sheats, Tacks, &c that it may not run out again till loos'd

A Bend, is the outwardmost Timber on the Ship's Side, and is also call'd a *Wale*. These are the chief Strength of the Ship's Side, to which the *Futtocks* and Knees of the Beams are made fast, and they are call'd the First, Second, &c beginning with that next the Water

Bent, or *to Bend*, us'd in the common Sense, as when the Shank of the Anchor is bow'd with overmuch ſtraining, they ſay, *It is bent* But the Uſe is different when they ſay, *Is the Cable bent?* which ſignifies, Is the Cable ſeas'd and made faſt to the Ring of the Anchor *Unbend the Cable*, that is, unbind it, and is done when they expect to be long at Sea, before they come to a Harbour

To bend Two Cables or *Ropes together*; is to tie them together with a Knot, and then make their own Ends faſt upon themſelves, which is not ſo ſure as ſplicing them together, but ſooner done, and moſt us'd, when it is deſign'd to take them aſunder again.

A Berth, is a convenient Diſtance, and Room to moor a Ship in And when they would go clear of a Point or a Rock they ſay, *Take a good Berth*; that is, go good Diſtance off to Sea from it

Berthing The riſing or bringing up of the Ship's Sides is call'd a Berthing So they ſay, A *Clincher* has her Sides Berth'd up, before any Beam be put into her

A Bight; is any Part of a Rope, as it is taken compaſſing, as when they cannot or will not take the End in Hand because of a Cable or other ſmall Rope being quoil'd up, they ſay, *Give me the Bight*, or, *Hold by the Bight*, that is, by one of the *Tacks*, which lie roul'd up one over the other

Bilboes, are Irons, or a kind of Stocks us'd aboard Ships for the Puniſhment of Offenders, and are more or leſs ponderous

ous, according to the Quality of the Of-
ence

Bildge, or *Buldge*, is the Breadth of the
loor, whereon the Ship rests, when she
a ground

Bildg'd, or *Buldg'd* A Ship is said to
e *Bildg'd* or *Buldg'd* when she strikes on
Rock, or an Anchor, or the like, and
eaks off her Timber or Planks there,
nd so springs a-Leak

Bildge Water, is the Water which, by rea-
n of the Ship's Breadth and Depth, cannot
ome to the Well, but lies in the Bildge

Bittacle, is a close Cupboard, plac'd in
e Steeridge, before the Whip or Tiller,
which the Compass stands, and is not
sten'd together with Iron Nails, but
ooden Pins, because Iron would draw
Needle, which would cause it never to
and true It is so contriv'd as to carry Can-
es in it, to give Light to the Compass,
d yet not to disperse any about the Ship.

A Bitter, is only a Turn of the Cable
out the Bitts, which is us'd in coming
an *Anchor* in any great Tide, Current,
Wind, especially in deep Water, when
e Cable is run out a convenient way,
en they give the Cable a Turn about
e Bitts, that they may veer it out at
le by little and little Else, if a Stop-
r should chance to fail, the Cable
uld run all out, or, as the Phrase is,
nd for End This Turn of the Cable is
ll'd a *Bitter*, and when the Ship is thus
opp'd, they say, *The Ship is brought up to
Bitter*

A Bit-

A Bitter End, is that End of the Ca which is uſually within Board, ſtill at t Bitts When the Ship rides at an A chor, ſo that when they would have th End bent to the Anchor, they ſay, Be *to the Bitter-End*

The Bitts, are the Two main ſqua Pieces of Timber which ſtand Pill wiſe, commonly plac'd abaft the Ma ger in the Loof of the Ship, for other Uſe but to belay the Cable to, wh the Ship rides at Anchor The low Part of them is faſten'd in *Hold* to t *Riders*, but the middle Part is bolted great Ships to Two Beams, which cro the Bows of the Ship, and therefore great Storms the Cable is ſometimes ma faſt to the Main-maſt to relieve the Bi and ſave the Bows

Blocks; are flattiſh oval Pieces of Woo with Sheevers in them, for all the ru ning Ropes to run in, and there are ſeve ral Sorts of them, as, ſingle Blocks, do ble Blocks, and ſome with Three, Fo and Five Sheevers in them, taking the Names from the Ropes they ſerve to, the Sheat-Block, the Tack-Block, th Fiſh-Block, *&c*

Blow This is a Word common to Men, but it is us'd ſome ways at Sea th are not generally underſtood, as, T *Wind blows home*, or *blows through*, that when it does not ceaſe, or grow leſs till comes paſt that Place *Blow through* alſo us'd, when they think the Wind wi so boisterous, that it will blow the ils asunder

Bluff, or *Bluff-headed*. When a Ship has mall Rake forward on, and so that she built with her Stem too streight up, is call'd *Bluff-headed*.

Board. Vide *Bord*.

Boat. The only Boat in a Ship call'd this Name is the Long Boat, which ust be able to carry out and weigh the t Anchor, and it will live in any a, unless it breaks very much. This t is reckon'd the very Model of a p being answerable to it in all its ts. The other Boats belonging to a p are, a Barge, a Pinnace, and a Skiff Shallop, which see in their Places.

A Bold Boat, is one that will endure a ugh Sea well.

Man the Boat, is, send Men in to row d steer it.

Fend the Boat, save her from beating nst the Ship's Side.

Wind the Boat, bring her Head the other y.

Boat the Anchor, put the Anchor into Boat.

The Boat-Rope, is the Rope by which Boat is tow'd at the Ship's Stern.

Boatswain. An Officer in a Ship who s Charge of all the Ropes belonging the Rigging of the Ship in general, all Cables and Anchors, all her Sails, her Flags, Colours and Pendants; and be answerable for them. He is also to take

take Care of the Long-Boat, and its Furniture, and either he or his Mate goes in and steers her upon all Occasions It is also his Duty to call up all the Men to their Watches, Spels and Work, and to see they perform them, and to keep the Peace among them And lastly, he is to see all Punishments inflicted on Offenders

Bolt, or *Bolts* Iron Pins us'd in the building and rigging of a Ship, whereof there are several Kinds, as *Ring-Bolts*, of great use for the bringing to of the Planks and Wales to the Ship, and for fastening the Tackles and Breechings of the Ordnance *Drive-Bolts*, which are long ones to drive out other Bolts or Trenels, u' in Building, for fixing the Planks and other Works together *Clench-Bolts* which are clench'd with a Riveting Hammer to prevent their drawing *Forelock-Bolts* which are made with an Eye at the End through which a Forelock of Iron is driven, to keep it from starting back *Fender Bolts*, made with a long Head, and beat into the outwardmost Bend of the Ship, to save her Sides, if another Ship should lie aboard her Bolts also take their Names from the Places where they are used, as Chain-Bolts, Bolts for Carriages, *&c* The Use of them is so great that a Ship cannot be built strong without them, because they bind all Parts together.

Bolt-Rope The Rope into which the Sail is sew'd, or made fast. It is a Three-stran

[...]trand Rope, not twisted so hard as others, [b]ut loose and soft, that it may ply the [b]etter to the Sail, and that the Sail may [b]e more easily sew'd into it

Bolt-sprit, is a Mast running out at the [H]ead of the Ship, not standing upright [a]s other Masts do, but lying along aslope [T]he But-End of it is generally set against [t]he Foot of the Fore-Mast, so that they [a]re a Stay to one another The Length [w]ithout Board is as much as may suffice [fo]r its Sail to hang clear of all Incum[b]rance. To this are fasten'd all the Stayes [th]at belong to the Fore-Mast, Fore-Top-[M]ast, and Fore-Topgallant-Mast, with [th]eir Boulings, Tacks, *&c* besides the [R]igging that belongs to its own particular [Sa]ils, which are only two, *viz* the Sprit-[sa]il, and Spritsail-Topsail. If the Bolt-[sp]rit fail in bad Weather, the Fore-Mast [ca]nnot hold long after; the Proportion of [th]em both is the same for Length and Big[n]ess

Bonaventure-Missen; is the Sternmost of [th]e Two, when a Ship happens to have [T]wo Missens, as some great Ships have [ha]d, but is now little us'd

Bonnet, is an additional Piece of Can[va]s to a Sail, to gather more Wind, and [co]mmonly us'd only to the Missen, Main, [F]oresail, and Spritsail Topsail Bon[ne]ts are very rare, though useful enough [in] an easie Gale The Depth of it is com[m]only One third of the Course it belongs [to], but there is nothing certain in these Cases,

Cases, for some make the *Main-Sail* exce[...] five deep, others much showler. No[...] That in speaking of the Sail with t[...] Bonnet, it is always call'd a Course, a[...] not a Sail, as Main-Course and Bonn[...] not Main-Sail, and so of the rest.

Lace on the Bonnet, or *bring to the Bonn[...]* is, put it to the Sail.

Shake off the Bonnet, is, take it off.

Boom, is a long Pole generally us'd [...] spread out the Clew of the Studding [...] yet sometimes the Clew of the Main-[...] and Fore-sail is boom'd out. Booms [...] also Poles with Bushes or Baskets on the[...] to shew Men how to see in the Chan[...] when a Country is overflown.

Booming; is stretching out the Clew of [...] Sail with the Boom, and is never us'd [...] upon Quarter-Winds, and before a Wi[...]

A Ship comes Booming, is, she comes w[...] all the Sail she can make.

Boord, or *Board*, is not only meant [...] Boards so call'd ashore, but *a-Boord* [...] *a-Board*, in the Sea Phrase, signifies wit[...] the Ship. To go a-Boord, is to go i[...] the Ship. *Bring the Tack close a-Boord*, [...] pull down the Tack close to the Chest[...] or the Gun Wale.

Boord and *Board*, is when Two Sh[...] lie Side by Side.

To make a-Boord, or, *To Boord it up* [...] *Place*, is to turn to Windward, stand[...] sometimes one Way, and sometimes [...] other, to gain to Windward.

A good Boord, is when there is m[...] gain'd to Windward.

To leave a Land on Back-Boord; is to leave it a-stern or behind the Back Boord, being that we lean our Backs against in Boats

To boord a Ship, is in Fight to come and lye so close as to touch the Enemy's Ship, that the Men may go out of the one into the other The best Place for Boording is the Bow, or athwart the Haws, and worst in the Quarter

Boomgrace, is a Frame or Composition of old Ropes, or Juncks of Cables, us'd to be laid out at the Bows, Stems and Sides of Ships, to preserve them from great Fleaks of Ice, when they sail far Northward or Southward.

Bouy Vide *Buoy*

The Bow, is the Part of the Ship that is broadest before, and begins at the Loof, and comes compassing about towards the Stem The due Proportion of this Part is of great Consequence for the Ship's sailing, because it breaks off the Sea, and is the Part which bears the Ship forward, being in a manner all the bearing of the Ship Now if the Bow be too broad, the Ship cannot make good Way through the Sea, because of the much dead Water before her, and if it be too lean or thin, she will pitch and beat extreamly, for want of Breadth to bear her up, so that there must be an exact Mean allow'd between them both

A Bold Bow, is a broad round Bow

A Lean Bow, is a narrow thin Bow

Lee

The Bow-Piece, is that which lies in th
Bow

Bowling, is a Rope that is fasten'd t the Leech, or middle Part of the outsi of the Sail, and the use of it is to mak a Sail stand sharper or closer by a Wind It is fasten'd to the Sail in two, three four, or more Places, which is call'd th Bowling-Bridle, only the Missen-Bowlin is fasten'd to the lower End of the Yard All Sails have this Rope, except the Sprit sail and Spritsail-Topsail, which have n Place to hale a Bowling forward by, an therefore cannot be us'd close by a Wind

Sharp the Main-Bowling, set taught th Bowling, hale up the Bowling, are all Term to pull it up hard, or more forward on.

Ease the Bowling, Check, or *Come up t Bowling*, is let it more slack.

Bowling-Bridle Vide *Bowling*

Bower; is an Anchor generally carri at the Ship's Bow, whence it has th Name, the greatest Anchor being for th most part in the Hould.

Bows, or *Bowse* This Word is us'd make Men pull together, but most by th Gunners, when they hale upon th Tackles, to thrust a Piece out of the Por

To brace a Yard, is to bring it to an one Side, and traverse it, that is, to s it any way over-thwart

Braces, are Ropes belonging to Yards, except the Missen They have Pendant, which is seaz'd to the Yar Arms, for there are Two Braces to ea

Yar

ard; and at the End of the Pendant a Block is seaz'd, through which the Rope is reev'd, which they call the Brace, the Use whereof is to square and traverse the Yards

Brackets, are little Pieces, in the Nature of Knees, which belong to the supporting of Galleries or Ship-heads

Brayls, are small Ropes reev'd through Blocks, which are seaz'd on either Side the Ties, some small Distance off upon the Yards, and so come down before the Sails, and are fasten'd to the Creengleys at the Skirt of the Sail The Use of them is to hale up the Bunt of the Sail when they farthel their Sails a-cross These Brayls belong only to the Two Courses, and to the Missen

Bread Room, is a Part of the Hould, separated by a Bulk-head from the rest, where the Bread and Bisket for the Men is kept

Breech, and *Breeching* The Breech is the aftermost Part of the Gun, from the Touch-hole; and the Ropes, which are bigger than the Tackles that make fast the Ordnance to the Ship's Side, being brought about the Breech of the Piece, are call'd *Breechings*, which are chiefly used in foul Weather

Brest-fast, is a Rope fasten'd to some Part of the Ship forward on, and so holds fast the Ship's-Head to a Wharf or other Place

Brest-

Brest-Ropes, are those which make fast the Parcel to the Yard

Brest-Hooks, are the compassing Timbers before, which help to fortify and strengthen the Ship's Stem, and all her fore Part

A Brest-Rope, is that which lashes the Parrel to the Mast

Bridle Vide *Bowling*

Brieze, is a Wind that blows out of the Sea, and daily keeps its Course in all seasonable Weather, beginning at a certain Hour in the Morning, and lasting till towards Night

Bring home the Anchor; is to weigh it.

Brooming, is when a Ship is brought aground, or on the Careen to be trimm'd, that is, to be made clean, then they burn off the old Weeds or Stuff, which has gather'd Filth, and this is usually done either with Reed, Broom, old Ropes or the like

Budge-Barrel, is a little Barrel, containing an Hundred Weight of Powder, and has a Leather Purse made fast at the End, which is to shut over the Powder, to keep it from Fire

Bucket The same as is us'd on Land to draw up Water

Bucket-Rope The Rope to which the Bucket is made fast to draw up Water

Bulk, is the whole Content of a Ship in Hould, or the Quantity of Goods it will stow for a Voyage.

To break Bulk, is to open the Hould. dispose of any of the Goods there

Bulk Head, is any Division made a cross Ship with Boards, to divide one Room m another, as the Bulk-head of the bin, the Bulk-head of the Half-Deck Bulk head of the Bread Room, the n Room, *&c*

Bunt, is as it were the Bag of a Sail, ch is allow'd in all Sails, that they receive much Wind If a Sail have much Bunt, it will hang too much Leeward, and hinder the Ship's sailing, cially by the Wind, and if it have little, then it will not hold Wind ough, and consequently not give the p sufficient Way This Difference is in the Top-sails, for Courses are cut re or with small Compass

Bunt-Lines, are small Lines, made fast the bottom of the Sails, in the middle t of the Bolt-Rope to a Creengle, and so reev'd through a small Block, d to the Yard, the Use whereof is ile up the Bunt of the Sail, for the ter fartheling and making of it up

Buoy, is a Piece of Wood, Barrel, or like which floats right over the Anchor, and is made fast by the Buoy Rope the Flook The Use whereof is not ly to shew where the Anchor is, but to weigh the Anchor with the Boat; ich is sooner done than with the Ship ere are other *Buoys*, which are left at chor in the Sea, to shew where there are

are Sands or Rocks; and these are mo useful where Sands remove, or whe there are no good Land Marks.

Buoyant, is any thing that floats

To buoy up a Cable, is to make fast a Piece of floating Wood, Barrel, or t like, to the Cable, somewhat near t Anchor, that the Cable may not tou the Ground: Used in foul Ground, whe they fear the cutting of the Cable

Stern the Buoy, that is, before they the Anchor fall, whilst the Ship has W they put the Buoy into the Water that the Buoy-Rope may be stretch'd o strait, that so the Anchor may fall cl from entangling it self with the Bu Rope

Burrel-Shot Vide *Case-Shot*

Burthen, is the Quantity of Goods Ship can stow; whence they say, she so many Tuns Burthen

Butt, generally taken for a Cask, a Butt of Wine, *&c* In the Sea-Langua a Butt is properly the End of a Pla joining to another on the outside o Ship, under Water

Butt-Heads, are the same, being the En of the Planks

To spring a Butt, is when a Plank is lo at one End

The Buttock; is the Breadth of the Sh right a-Stern, from the Tuck upward

C

C

CAble, is a Three-ſtrand Rope, of a ſuitable Strength and Bigneſs for Ship to ride by at an Anchor, which herwiſe is counted but a Hawſer; for great Ship's Hawſer will make a ſmaller hip's Cable *Cables* have their ſeveral ppellations, as the Anchors have, being ll'd the Firſt, Second, Third, beginning ith the laſt, till you come to the *Sheet*-nchor-Cable

To lay a Cable, is to make a Cable

Sarve, or plat the Cable, is to bind me old Ropes or Clouts about it, to e it from gauling the Hawſe

To ſplice a Cable; is to interweave and ſten two Ends of it together

To quoile the Cable; is to lay it up in owls one upon another

Cable Tire, is the Cable ſo laid up in owls

To pay more Cable, is to heave out more Sea from the Ship.

To pay Cheap; is to throw it over

To veer more Cable; is to let it run out.

Shot of Cable Vide *Shot*

Caburn; is a ſmall Line, made of ſpun rn, to bind the Cables, or to make a nd of Two Cables, or to ſeaze the inding-Tacks, or the like

Calm, is when there is no Wind at , to which Word are added theſe Epi-ets, flat, dead, or ſtark Calm *Becalming* to be ſeen in its Place

K C*am*-

Cambering, or to Camber A Deck is said to lie *Cambering*, when it is higher in the Middle than at either End: And the Word is commonly apply'd to the Ship's Keel and Beams, and other rounding Pieces of the Ship's Frame.

Camber-Keel'd, is when the Keel is bent in the Middle upwards, which may be occasion'd by her lying ashore, when her Ends do not touch, and by other Accidents

Cantique-Quoins. Vide *Quoins*

The Cap, is the square Piece of Timber put over the Head of any Mast, with a round Hole in it, to receive the Top mast into it, or Flag-staff, by which the Top mast is kept steddy Every Mast has a Cap if it carries another, or but a Flag-staff at the Top

Cap-Squares, are the broad Pieces of Iron which belong to either Side of the Carriage of a Gun, to look over the Trunnions of the Piece, over which they are made fast in an Iron Pin with a Fore-lock. The *Use* of them is to keep the Gun from flying out of the Carriage, when fir'd, the Mouth of it lying very low, or under Metal.

Capstam There are Two of them, the Main-Capstain, and the Jeer-Capstain. The Main-Capstain is that Piece of Timber which is plac'd upright next behind the Main-mast, the Foot of it standing in a Step on the lower Deck, and the Head betwixt the Two upper Decks. The Pa

Parts of this Capſtain are the Foot, which is the longeſt Part, the *Spindle*, being its ſmalleſt Part, the *Whelps* which are like Brackets ſet upon the Body of the *Capſtain*, cloſe under the Bars, the *Barrel*, which is the main Subſtance, or Poſt of the whole Piece, the Holes for the Bars to be put into; the *Bars*, which are ſmall Pieces of Timber, whereby the Men heave, that is, turn it round, and the *Pawl*, being a Piece of Iron bolted to one End of the Beams of the Deck, cloſe to the Body of the Capſtain, yet ſo that it has Liberty to turn about every way, and againſt it the Whelps of the Capſtain do ſo bear, that it may be ſtopp'd from turning or reverſing upon Occaſion; which Stoppage is call'd, Pawling of the Capſtain. The Uſe of the Capſtain is to weigh the Anchors, to hoiſe or ſtrike down the Top maſts, to heave into the Ship any thing of great Weight, or to ſtrain a Rope that requires much Force The *Jeer-Capſtain* is plac'd in the ſame manner between the Fore and Main-maſts, the Uſe whereof is to heave upon the Jeer-Rope, or to hold off when the Anchor is weighing At the Foot of it are alſo Whelps, but leſs than thoſe of the Firſt, which ſerve to heave upon the *Viol*, for the Help of the Main-Capſtain, in weighing a great Anchor The Terms us'd at it are, *Come up Capſtain*, that is, thoſe at the Capſtain muſt go backward, and ſlacken the Rope or Cable which they heave at *Launch at th Capstain*, is heave no more *Pawl the Capstain*, that is, stay, or stop it with the Pawl, which bears against the Whelps, to keep it from running round, back, or reversing

Capstain-Bars, are small Pieces of Timber put through the Barrel of the Capstain through square Holes, of equal Length on both Sides, by which the Men heave and turn about the Capstain

Capstain Punishment, is when a Capstain Bar being thrust through the Hole of the Barrel, the Offender's Arms are extended at the full Length Cross-wise, and so ty'd to the Bar, having sometimes a Basket of Bullets, or other heavy Thing, hanging at his Neck, which he is to endure according to the Nature of the Offence

Captain, is the Commander in Chief aboard any Ship of War, for those in Merchants are improperly call'd so, having no Commissions, and being only Masters. The Captains ought always to be Men of consummate Experience, and try'd Valour

Careen, or *Careening*, is the best Way of trimming a Ship under Water both in regard that the Carpenters may stand upon Scaffolds commodiously to caulk the Seams, or do what else is requisite and for firing of the Ground Timbers This Careening is to be done in Harbours where the slower the Tide runs, the better; and it is most us'd where there are no Docks to trim Ships in, nor conve-
nien

ient Place to grave them on, or that it
does not ebb so much as for a Ship to
shew dry The Manner of Careening is
this, They take out all, or leave but very
little of the Provision, Ballast, Ordnance,
or the like, in the Ship, and there
must be a lower Ship by her, with which
she must be laden down to a Side, and
righted again with Tackles, but they rather
effect it with the Weight of Ballast
above or below, and so never strain the
Masts much

Carlings, are those Timbers which lie along the Ship, from one Beam to another, and serve not only to strengthen the Ship, but on them the Ledges rest, to which the Planks of the Deck are fasten'd

Carling-Knees; are those Timbers which come a-thwart Ships from the Ship's Side to the *Hatch-way*, which is betwixt the Two Masts They bear the Deck on them on both Sides the Mast, and on the Ends of the Coomings lie the Hatches

Carnel-Work The first building of Ships with their Timbers and Beams, and after bringing on their Planks, to distinguish it from *Clinch-Work*

Carpenter, is either a Ship-Carpenter to build a Ship, or one aboard a Ship to keep her in Repair

A Carriage; is that whereon a Gun is mounted, the Parts whereof are, the Two *Cheeks*, the *Axletrees*, the *Bolts*, the *Cap squares*, the *Hooks*, the *Forelocks*, the

 Trucks,

Trucks, and the *Linse Pins* See each of them in its proper Place

Cartridge, is a Bag of Canvas, or a Roll of Paper or Parchment, made upon a Former, the Diameter whereof must be somewhat smaller than the Cylinder of the Piece, and of such Length as will contain as much Powder as is the Charge of the Piece, being absolutely necessary for speedy lading, and to avoid the Danger of firing loose Powder The best Cartridges are those of Parchment, because they leave no Fire in the Piece when discharg'd

Cartridge-Cases, are made of Tin, to carry the Cartridges in for fear of firing

Carvels, are Vessels which use Mizzen Sails instead of Main-Sails They will lie nearer the Wind than Cross-Sails but are not so commodious for handling and not us'd at all in *England*

Case; is commonly made round of Wood, and hollow, fit for the Bore of a Piece, to charge it with murdering, that is, small Shot Bags are also us'd for this Purpose, but are not so convenient because they are apt to catch hold in the Flaws of the Piece

Case-Shot, is any old Iron, Stones, Musket-Bullets, or the like, which they put into Cases to shoot out of great Guns and makes great Havock among Men and Ships come near, or lie Board and Board

Casing a Ship, is sometimes us'd for *Sheathing* of her

Caskets, are small Strings made of Sinnet-Flat. They are made fast to the upper Part of the Yards, in little Rings, called Grommets Their Use is to make fast the Sail to the Yard, when they farthel it up The biggest and longest are plac'd just in the Middle of the Yard, betwixt the Ties, to make up the Bunt of the Sail, and are call'd *Brest-Caskets*

Catherpins; are small Ropes, running in little Blocks from one Side of the Shrowds to the other, near the Deck, to keep the Shrowds taught for the better Ease and Safety of the Mast in the rowling of the Ship, and only us'd to the Main and Fore Shrowds.

Cat; is a Piece of Timber fasten'd aloft, right over the Hawse, and at one End of it has Two Sheevers, wherein is a Rope, with a Block, to which is fasten'd a great Iron Hook · The Use is to trise up the Anchor from the Hawse to the Top of the Forecastle, where it is fasten'd with a Stopper

Cat the Anchor; is to hitch the Hook in the Ring of the Anchor

Cat-Holes, are Two little Holes a-Stern, above the Gun-Room Ports, to bring in a Cable or Hawser through them to the Capstain, when there is Occasion to heave the Ship a-Stern by a Stern Fast; the Stern-Ports being not so proper for this Purpose, because they do not lie so even with the Capstain

Caulk, or *Caulking*, is driving of Oakham, or the like, into the Seams, Rends and Treenels throughout the Ship, without which she cannot be tight to keep out Water.

Chafe, or *Chafing*; is when a Rope gawles or frets against any thing that is too hard for it, or that is not smooth and even.

Chains, in a Ship, signify those Chains to which the Shrows are made fast on the Ship's Sides; and those belonging to the Top-mast Shrowds. In Fight, the Yards are slung in Chains, lest the Ties should be cut, and the Yards fall, which Chains are call'd Slings.

Chain-Walls; is a broad Timber set on the outside of the Ship, on purpose to spread out the Shrowds wider, that they may the better ease the Mast.

A Chamber, is a Charge of Brass or Iron, us'd to be put in at the Breech of any Murderer, containing as much Powder as is requisite to deliver out the Case-Shot contain'd in the Piece. The Chamber of a Gun, is that Part of it that contains the Charge.

Channel; is the deepest Part of any River, or Harbour's-Mouth, and where the greatest Current of Water is. Narrow Seas are sometimes call'd Channels, as the *English* Channel between *France* and *England*, and St. *George*'s Channel between *England* and *Ireland*.

Charge, is as much Powder and Shot as belongs to any Piece. At Sea they say, Charge a Musket, but load or lade a great Gun. A Ship of great Charge is generally one that draws much Water. Every Man's Office aboard a Ship is alſo call'd his Charge.

Chaſe, when any Ship makes all the Sail ſhe can to fetch up another, it is call'd Chaſing, and the Ship ſo purſu'd is call'd the *Chaſe*. *A-Stern Chaſe*, is when one Ship follows another right a-Stern.

Chaſe-Pieces, are thoſe which lie as well right aft, as right forward; the latter ſerving upon chaſing another, and the former when chas'd.

The Ship has a good Chaſe, is meant of her Chaſe forwards, that is, when ſhe is built to carry ſeveral Guns to point juſt forward. In the other Caſe they ſay, *A-Stern Chaſe*.

Checks, are two Pieces of Timber, fitted on each Side of the Maſt, from beneath the Hounds to the uppermoſt End of the Maſt. They are made of Oak, to ſtrengthen the Maſt thereabouts, both for bearing of the Top-maſt, and hoiſing of the Yards. The Knees that faſten the Beak-Head to the Bow of the Ship, are alſo call'd *Cheeks*; ſo are the Sides of any Blocks, as alſo the Sides of the Carriages, where the Trunions of the Pieces lie.

Cheſtrees, are two ſmall Pieces of Timber, with a Hole in them, the one on the one Side of the Ship and the other on the other Side; through which Holes the Main-Tack runs. They are plac'd a little abaft the Loof the Ship

Choak When a running Rope sticks in the Block, either by slipping betwixt the Cheeks and the Sheever, or any other Accident, so that it cannot run, they say, The Block is choak'd

Clamps, are the thick Timbers lying fore and aft, close under the Beams of the first *Orlop* Vide *Risings*

A Cleat; is a small Wedge of Wood, fasten'd on the Yards, to keep any Ropes from slipping by where it is fasten'd, and for other Uses, as to keep the Eating of the Sail from slipping off the Yard. There are also Cleats made fast in several Places, being small Bits of Wood to belay the Ropes to

Clench-Bolts Vide *Bolts*

The Clew, is the lower Corner of the Sail, which reaches down to the Part where the Tacks and Sheets are made fast to the Sail, and is that Part which comes goaring down out from the Square of the Sail towards the lower Corner

Clew-Garnet; is a Rope made fast to the Clew of the Sail, and running thence in a Block, which is seaz'd to the Middle of the Yard The Use of it, in farthelling up the Main-Sail, or Fore-Sail

Clew-Line, is the same to Top, Top Gallant and Spritsails that the Clew-Garnet is to the Main-Sail, and has the very same Use.

Clincher; is a small Ship, Bark or Boat, whose Planks and Boards are larded over one another, and clench'd and nail'd through one another with Nails and Rooves; whose Outsides are berth'd or wrought up without Timber, fram'd as we do in other Ships, which Work is call'd *Carvel Work*

To Clinch, is to batter or rivet a Bolt's-End upon a Ring, or to turn back the Point of a Nail, that it may hold fast

The Clinch of the Cable; is that of it which is seaz'd about the Ring of the Anchor

Clinching, is a sort of slight caulking, us'd at Sea when the Water beats in at the Ports, then the Carpenter is commanded to *Clinch the Ports*, which is to drive a little Ockham into the Seams of them

Cloath A Sail is said to cloath the Mast, when it is so long, that it touches the Gratings or Hatches, so that no Wind can get betwixt them and it

Close upon a Tack, or *Close by a Wind*, is when the Wind is almost a-head, and the Sails-Clews are carry'd forwards, that they may take the Wind to make the best of their Way

Cloth. They say, a Ship spreads much Cloth when she has broad Sails

Cloy'd When any thing is got into the Touch-hole or Breech of the Piece, so

that

that the Priming-Powder cannot come to give Fire to the rest, they say, The Piece is cloy'd.

Coamings, or *Coaming of the Hatche*, or *Gratings*; is that Piece of Timber or Plank which bears them up higher than the Decks; the Use of them being to keep the Water from running down the Hatches.

Coats, are the Pieces of Tarr'd Canvas which are put above the Masts at the Partners, and the Lumps at the Deck, that no Water may run down by them The same is us'd at the Rudder-Head

Cock-bell When the Cable hangs right up and down by the Ship's Side, it is said to be a Cock-bell.

Cock-Boat; is the smallest sort of Boat, and of very little Service at Sea

Cocks; are little square Rings of Brass, put into the middle of the greatest Wooden Sheaves, to keep them from splitting by the Pin of the Block whereon they turn.

Cockswain; is an Officer who is to have Care of the Barge or Shallop, and all Things thereto belonging, and to command the Men that man the Boat upon all Occasions; and is therefore allow'd to carry a Whistle

Collar, is the Rope that is made fast about the Beak-Head, to which the Dead-Man's-Eye is seaz'd, to which the Main Stay is fasten'd There is also a Rope about the Main-Mast-Head which is called d a Collar, or a Garland, plac'd there to ve the Shrowds from gawling

The Comb, is a small Piece of Timber t under the lower Part of the Beak-Head, near the midst, with two Holes in, and has the same Use to the Fore-Tacks that the *Chesstrees* have to the Main-Tacks, which is, to bring the Tack board

Come up Capstain Vide *Capstain*

Compass, is that movable Instrument ith a Fly, whereon are describ'd the Points or Winds they steer by at Sea. is in a round Box, close cover'd with Glass, the Fly hanging on a Point, and uch'd to the Loadstone, which makes always point to the North

To Cond, or *Con*, is to direct the Man at e Helm how to steer, which is done by e standing on the Deck

In Consort, is, Ships sailing together in ompany

Cook His Office at Sea is the same as shore

Cook-Room; is the Place where the Meat dress'd

Cordage, is all kind of Ropes belonging the Rigging of a Ship

Corn-Powder Vide *Powder*

Corporal His Office at Sea is to look all the small Arms, and keep them 'd and clean, their Bandaleers fill'd with Powder, and to exercise such as are pointed to use Muskets in Fight

Coun-

Counter, is the hollow Arching Part the Ship's Stern, betwixt the Transf and the lower Part of the Gallery, whi is call'd the *Lower Counter* The *Up Counter* is from the Gallery to the low Part of the Upright of the Stern

Course; is that Point of the Comp the Ship is to sail upon

A Course, is also a Sail, as, the *Ma Course* and *Fore-Course*, which are, the Fo Sail and Mizzen-Sail without Bonnets

Courteaux, very short great Guns, sca us'd at this Time

Crab, is an Engine of Wood, wi three Claws plac'd on the Ground, in t Nature of a Capstain, most common us'd where they build Ships for launchi out, or heaving in a Ship into the Doc

Cradle, is a Frame of Timber broug along the outside of a Ship by a Bildg wherein they launch Ships for the great Safety

Craft, is any kind of Nets, Lines, Hooks to catch Fish Small Vessels, Hoys, Ketches, and the like, are al call'd *Small-Craft*

Crank A Ship is said to be Cran sided when she will bear but small Sa and lie down very much with little Win They also say, she is Crank by the Groun when she cannot be brought agroun but with Danger of overthrowing.

Creengles, are little Ropes splic'd in the *Bolt-Ropes* of all Sails belonging to t Main and Fore-mast, to which the *Bo lin*

ug *Bridles* are made fast, and they are llo to hold by when they shake off a lonnet.

Cross-Bar, is round Shot, with a Bar f Iron, as it were, put through the Midle, and sticking out at both Ends 6 or Inches, more or less, us'd in Fight for utting or spoiling of Ropes, Sails, Yards, nd Masts, and to do Execution among llen

Cross-Jack; is a Yard at the upper End f the Mizzen-Mast, under the Top, here it is flung, having no Halliards or Ties belonging to it The Use of it s to spread and hale on the Mizzen-Topail Sheets

Cross Piece; is the great Piece of Timer which goes a-cross the *Bit-Pipes*, and s that whereon they belay the Cable.

Cross-Trees, are those cross Pieces of Timber which are set on the Head of the Mast, bolted and let into one another vey strong All these Four Pieces are generally call'd Cross-Trees, but in Strictess, the Name belongs only to those Two which go athwart Ships; and the ther Two which go alongst Ships are all'd *Tressel-Trees* The Use of them is o keep the Top-Mast up, the Foot of the Top-Mast being fasten'd in them, so that hey bear all the Stress They also bear he Tops on them

Crows-Feet; are those small Lines or opes which stand in 6, 8, 10, or more arts, so divided and put through the Holes

Holes of a Dead-Man's-Eye, that the are of no Use, but only set up by th Boatswains to make the Ship shew full o small Rigging, and all plac'd to the Bot tom of the Back-Stays of the Fore-Top Mast, Spritsail Top-Mast, Mizzen Top Mast, and the Top-Gallant-Masts

Cubbridge-Head, is the same as a Bulk Head, only that this Word is us'd to th Bulk-Head of the Fore-Castle and th Half-Deck, which are call'd, the *Cub bridge-Head afore*, and the *Cubbridge Hea abaft*

Culver-Tail, is the Way of letting on Timber into another, so that they can n Way slip out

Cut When a Sail is well fashion'd they say, it is well Cut

Cut the Sail, is for the Men, when the are upon the Yard, to let it fall down

Cut the Cable, is when a Ship rides i a Storm, and must set Sail, but canno stay to weigh the Anchor

Cut the Mast by the Board, is done i great Storms

Cut-Water; is the Sharpness of the Sh before, which cuts the Water, and di vides it before it comes to the Bow

The Cylinder of a Gun; is the Bore o hollow Part of it, which receives th Charge

D

D*Avit*, is a Piece of Timber with a Notch at one End, to which they ...ng a Block by a Strap, call'd the Fish-...lock, by which they hale up the Flook ...f the Anchor to the Ship's Bow or ...oof It is not made fast to the Ship, ...ut shifted to either Side, as there is Oc-...sion; laid by till us'd, and then put ...ut betwixt the Cat and the Loof The ...ong Boat has a *Davit*, which is set over ...e Head of the Boat, with a Sheever, in-... which they bring the *Buoy-Rope* to ...igh the Anchor, and it stands in the ...rlings that are in the Boat's Bow ...unch *out*, or *Launch in the Davit*; is, ...t it out or in

Dead-Mens-Eyes; are a kind of Blocks ... which there are many Holes, but no ...eevers, through which the *Lanniers* go ...at make fast the Shrowds to the Chains. ...he Crows-Feet reeve through Dead-...ens-Eyes

Dead-Reckoning, is the Calculation they ...ake at Sea of the Place they are in, by ...mputing their several Runs upon dif-...ent Points, and setting them off on a ...per, so as to make a Judgment of the ...ace they are come to by their sailing, ...hen they cannot take an Observation.

Dead-Rope, is any Rope that does not ...n in a Block, but is us'd by Hand

Dead-

Dead-Water, is the Eddy Water at t Stern of the Ship, ſo call'd, becauſe does not paſs away with that Life a Quickneſs as the other does They ſ *A Ship holds much Dead-Water*; that is, a great Eddy follows her at the Stern Rudder

Deck, is the Floor of Planks where the Ordnance is plac'd, and the Men w and lye upon the Beams · They are ca the Firſt, Second, and Third Decks, ginning at the lowermoſt There is a the Half-Deck, being the Deck which from the Main-Maſt to the Stem Quarter-Deck, is from the Steeridge a to the Maſter's Cabbin. The Spar-De is the uppermoſt betwixt the Two Ma All theſe Decks are alſo call'd Orlops. Fluſh-Deck, is when it lies upon a L from Stem to Stern, without any R The Deck *Cambers*; is, when it does lie flat, but compaſſing To ſink, or let fall a Deck, is to place it lower. raiſe a Deck, is to place it higher abo Water

Deep-Sea-Lead, is the Lead that is ho at the *Deep-Sea-Line*, to ſink it down; Weight of it commonly 14 Pounds the Bottom of it is ſtuck ſome hard wh Tallow, which brings up the Grou and by the Difference of it they kn upon what Coaſt they are, but in ow Ground, they uſe a white Woollen Clo with a little Tallow, for without Cloth, the Owze would not ſtick to Tallow.

D

Deep-Sea-Line; a small Line, us'd in deep Waters to sound for finding Ground

To Disembogue; is to come out of the Mouth of any Gulph, which being large within, may have a strait and narrow coming out, but this is not us'd for going out of Harbour, or the like Occasions

To dispert, is to find out the Difference of the Diameters of the Metals between the Breech and the Mouth of any Piece of Ordnance, by which they know what Allowance to give to the Mouth of the Piece, being ever less than the Breech, that thereby they may make a true Shot. There are several Ways of doing it; but the easiest and best is to put in a Straw or small Stick at the Touch-hole, and then applying it in the same Manner to the Mouth, which will exactly shew the Difference of the Thickness of the Metal at the Breech and at the Mouth of the Piece

Dock. There are two Sorts of Docks; *Dry Dock*, which is made with Flood-Gates to keep out the Tide, in which Ships are built and repair'd, and where they sit without Danger or Harm, and a *Wet Dock*, being any Creek or Place where a Ship may be cast in out of the Tide's Way on the Owze When a Ship has there made her self a Place to lie in, they say, she has Dock'd her self

To Dock her self Vide *Dock*

A Drabler Vide *Bonnet*, for it is in all Respects to the Bonnet, as the Bonnet is

to

to the Course, being another Piece adde to it, and therefore only us'd when th Course and Bonnet are too showl to choa the Mast

Draggs All Things that hang over th Ship in the Sea, as Shirts, Gowns, or th like, as also the Boat in that Respect All hindering the Ship's Way under Sai are call'd *Draggs*

Drakes Small Guns, now little us'd Sea

Draught By the Draught of Water, meant so many Foot as the Ship goes i the Water, that is, the Part of her whic is under Water The greatest Men War draw 22 Foot Water.

To Dregg, or *Dregging*, is to take a li tle Grapnel, which being hung over th Boat's Stern, is let down to drag on th Ground, to find a Cable that has been l slip, to whose Anchor there was no Buoy for this being drawn along the Groun will take hold if it meets with it

A Drift-Sail, is a Sail us'd under Wa ter, being veer'd out right a-head wit Sheats to it; the Use whereof is to kee a Ship's Head right upon the Sea in Storm It is also good when a Shi drives in fast with the Current, to sto her driving so fast

Drive They say a Ship drives, whe the Anchor will not hold her fast, bu that she falls away with the Tide o Wind Also when a Ship is *a-Hull*, o *a-Trie*, they say, she drives to Leeward, in with the Shore, or the like.

Dr

Duck up; is a Term us'd with the Clew-Garnet and Clew-Lines of the Main-Sail, Fore Sail, and Sprit-Sail, when the two first Sails hinder his Sight forwards that steers Conds, and to the Sprit-Sail, when they fire the Chase-Guns, because the Clew of the Sprit-Sail will hinder the Sight

Ducking, is letting an Offender fall into the Sea two or three times with a Rope under his Arms, about his Middle, and under his Breech, from the Yard-Arm, which is a sort of Punishment us'd at Sea

E.

EAring, is that Piece or Part of the Bolt Rope which is left open at all the four Corners of the Sail, like a Ring the two uppermost are put over the Ends of the Yards or Yard-Arms, and the Sail is at those two Ends made fast to the Yard Into the lowermost the Tacks and Sheats are seaz'd, or, as the proper Term is, bent unto the Clew

To Ease, is to let any Rope slacker, and us'd to them all except the Tack; which, when to be slacken'd, they say, *Rise the Tack*, because it rises from the Chesstrees, to which it is hal'd close

Ease the Helm, is to let the Ship go more large, or right before the Wind

An Eddy, is the running back of the Water in any Place, contrary to the Tide, and so falling into the Tide again, occasion'd by some Head-Land or Point in a River, which stops the running of the Water.

An

An Eddy Wind, is that which recoils, returns back from any Sail, or the li going contrary to that Wind from whi it proceeded, but is never so strong

End for End, signifies a Rope being run out of the Block, so that it is u reev'd, or when the Cable or Hawse ru all out at the Hawse, signifying that it all gone to the End

To Enter; is to come into a Ship, es cially us'd in Boarding a Ship in Fight.

Entring-Ladders There are two of the the one us'd by the Ship's Side in Harbo and fair Weather, with Entring-Ropes it, which is all made of Wood. T other is of Ropes, with small Staves Steps, which is hung over the Galle for entring out of the Boat in foul W ther, when, by Reason of the Ship's h ving and setting, they dare not bring Boat to the Ship's Side for Fear of stavi

Entring-Rope, is the Rope that hangs the Side of the Ship, in the Waste, wh Men usually come aboard out of the Bo and taken generally for any Rope give Man to enter by

Eyes The Hole wherein the Ring the Anchor is put, is call'd the *Eye*, also the Compass or Ring, which is left the Strap to which a Block is seaz'd, led, the Eye of the Strap

Eyelet-Holes, are the round Holes al the Bottom of the Sails, which have B nets belonging to them, and *Bonnets* h the same for their Drablers. They all Line sown about them for more ength, and serve to receive the Latches the Bonnets or Drablers, with which Bonnet is lac'd to the Course, and the bler to the Bonnet

F

Faddom, is six Foot, by which all Ropes are measur'd

Faddom, is to measure by Faddoms, n sounding to find how deep the Water is

Fack; is one Circle of any Rope or ble that is quoil'd up round

The *Fall*; is that Part of the Rope of ickle which is haled upon.

Fall off, signifies that a Ship under l does not keep so near the Wind as directed.

Falls, signify the Rising or Falling of e Parts of the Deck

False-Keel, when a Ship rowls too much, reason that she is over-floating A Se- nd Keel is sometimes put under the st, and that is call'd, a False Keel

False-Sheat, is a Rope bound to the ew of the Sail, above the Sheat-Block, extraordinary Gusts, and very stiff les, to ease the Sheat, lest it should eak

To Farthel; is to wrap up a Sail close to- ther, and so bind it with Caskets to the rd, but towards the Yard they use ope-Yarns, because it is not there heavy

Far-

Furthelling-Lines, are small Lines mad fast to all the Top-Sails, Topgallant-Sail and the Mizzen-Yard-Arm The Mizz has but one, the other one on each Sid By these they furthel up those Sails, bu the Top-Sails have not their Bunt boun up to the Yard, as the Main and For Sails have, but it is laid on the Top, an so bound fast to the Head of the M which is call'd, *Stowing the Top-Sail*

Fashion-Pieces, are the two outermo Timbers of the Ship's Stern on eith Side, which shew the Breadth of the Sh there

Feazing, is ravelling out, as when Rope wears, and the Oakham ravels ou

To Fend the Boat, is to save her fro beating against the Rocks, the Shore, the Ship's Side

Fender-Bolts Vide *Bolts*

Fenders, are Pieces of old Cables, Rop or Billets of Wood, hung over the Shi Side, to keep another Ship or Boat fro rubbing against her, that they may n break her Bends, or rub off the St when she is new trimm'd Boats ha Fenders to keep them from beating agai the Ship's Side, and in the Boat the M have also short Staves, which they c *Fenders*, being for the same Use

Fetch home an Anchor Vide *Bring hom*

The Fidd, is an Iron Pin, made taper and sharp at the lower End, to open t Strands of the Ropes, when they spli two together. The Pin in the Heel the Top Maſt, which bears up the *Cheſs-Trees*, is alſo call'd a Fidd.

Fids, are in the ſame Nature as the Fidds, but made of Wood, pointed at the End, and larger, to open the Strands of Cables to ſplice them, and made of Wood because of Iron they would be too heavy to work with.

Fid Hammer, is a Fidd, as above, made ſharp at one End, to ſplice a Rope, and a Hammer at the other End, with a Head and a Claw, to drive or draw a Nail.

Fights. The waſte Cloths that hang about the Ship, to hinder Men from being ſeen in Fight, are call'd the *Fights*; the Bulk-Head afore and abaft, or any other Places where Men may cover themſelves, and make a Defence, are call'd, *Cloſe Fights*.

Fireworks, are any Sort of artificial Fire, apply'd to any Weapon or Inſtrument to fire the Hulls, Sails, or Maſts of Ships, in Fight, the commoneſt whereof at Sea are Fire Pots, Fire-Balls, Fire Peeks, Trunks, Braſs Balls, Arrows with Fire-works, &c.

A Fiſh, is any Piece of Timber or Plank made faſt to the Maſt or Yard, to ſtrengthen it, when in Danger of breaking.

The Fiſh, is a Tackle hung at the End of the *Davit*, by the Strap of the Block; to which Block there is a Runner, with a Hook at the End, which does hitch the Flook of the Anchor, ſo they hale by

 the

the Fall that belongs to it, and raise th Flook to the Bow, or *Chain-Wale* of th Ship

The Fish-Block, is the Block that belong to the Fish above describ'd

The Fish-Hook, is the Hook belonging t the Fish, as above

To Fish the Mast, or *the Yard*, is to pu a Piece of Timber or Plank to it, whe it is weak, to strengthen it, as was sa under the Word, *a Fish*

Flaggs, are us'd at Sea for Distincti of Nations and Commands, so the A miral has his at the Main-Top, the Vi Admiral in the Fore, and the Rear-Adm ral in the Mizzen-Top They are al us'd for Signals to direct Ships what th are to do, as to chase, to give over, come to Council, *&c* To strike the F in Fight, is a Token of yielding, oth wise it denotes paying Respect, and t Striking is pulling it down upon the C and to let it hang loose over

Flair When a Ship is hollow'd near the Water, so that the Work ha over, and is laid out broader aloft, th say, *The Work does Flair over*

To Flat in the Sail, is to pull the S flat by the Sheat, as near to the Shi Side as may be.

Flood. When the Water begins to r it is Flood. Quarter-Flood and H Flood are well known to signify the Ti being a quarter or half in

The Flook; is the broad Part of the

or which takes hold in the Ground, and of the Grapnels, which have four hooks. Vide *Anchor*.

The Floor, is as much of the Ship's Bottom as she rests upon when aground.

To Flote, is to swim above Water, but meant of inanimate Things which bear up naturally without helping themselves, *The Ship is a Flote*, that is, she is born up by the Water.

Floty. A Ship that draws little Water, is called Floty.

Flow. When the Water rises upon the coming in of the Tide, they say, it flows.

Flown. When any of the Sheats are not hal'd home to the Blocks, they say, *the Sheat is flown*, whence they also say, the Ship sails with Flown Sheats.

The Fly, is that Part of the Compass on which the 32 Points or Winds are described. To it the Needle touch'd to the Loadstone is made fast underneath, and always turns to the North.

To let Fly, is to let go a-main, or all at once, and as far as it will.

The Forecastle, is that Part of the Ship where the *Fore-Mast* stands, and is sever'd from the rest of the Floor by a Bulk-head.

Forefoot. There is no Place in a Ship that bears this Name, but when they say, one Ship lies with the Forefoot of the other, it signifies, That the one does lie with her Stem so much a-Weather the other, that keeping their Courses, she that lies so will go out a-head with the other, which

which is, one Ship's sailing a-cross an-other Ship's Way.

Forelocks, are little flat Pieces of Iron like Wedges, to put into the Holes at the Ends of Bolts, to keep them from draw-ing out, or slipping back.

Forelock-Bolts. Vide *Bolts*.

Fore-Mast. Vide *Mast*.

A Former, is a Piece of Wood turn'd round, somewhat less than the Bore of the Piece for which it is made; as, a Sa-ker-Former, a *Minion Former*, &c. The U[se] of it is, to make on it Linen, Paper [or] Parchment Cartridges for the Guns.

Fore-Reach. When two Ships sail toge-ther, or after one another, she that sa[ils] best, that is, fastest, is said to Fore-rea[ch] upon the other.

Fore-Sail. Vide *Sail*.

Fore-Top-Mast. Vide *Mast*.

Fore-Yard. Vide *Yard*.

Foul. When a Ship has been long u[n]trimm'd, so that Grass or any other Thi[ng] grows or sticks about her, she is said to [be] foul. Also when any Rope is so tang[led] or stopp'd by any Accident whatsoev[er] that it cannot run, it is said to be foul.

Foul-Water. When a Ship under S[ail] comes into shallow Water, so that she [rai-] ses the Mud or Sand with her Way, [as] she may do without touching the Grou[nd] but only coming very near it, they [say] *she makes foul Water*.

To Founder, is when a Ship, by an ex-traordinary Leak, or some gre[at] broken into her is full, or half ful Water, so that it cannot be deliver'd , and then like a founder'd Horse she not go, nor will she feel her Helm, drive in the Sea like a Log of Wood, ich generally sinks her, and therefore hen a Ship is lost out at Sea, the com- Expression is, *She founder'd at Sea*

Freight, is the Burthen of Goods put into a Ship, and thence the Price paid the Carriage of those Goods, accor- ng to the Bulk or Weight, and the D- ance of the Place

To Free the Ship, is to get the Water of her, and so, to free the Boat, sig- fies the same Thing And this Word is t us'd to any other Purpose about the ip

Fresh-Shot When any extraordinary Wa- r comes down a River suddenly from e Land, or when a very great River car- es its fresh Water a Mile or two into e Sea, they say, It is a great fresh Shot

Fresh the Hawse, is, let out a little more ble at the Hawse, that a fresh Part may ome to endure the Stress, and not fret e Place altogether.

Furling-Lines, are those small Lines ade fast to all the Top-Sails, Topgallant- ails, and the Mizzen-Yard Arms, of hich the Mizzen has but one, and the thers one on each Side, the Use of them eing to *furl* that is, to gather up the ls

To Furl the Sails, is to gather them u close, and bind them fast about the Yard

Fur, or *Furr'd* There are two Sorts o Furring, the one is, after a Ship is buil to lay on another Plank upon the Side o her, which is call'd, *Plank upon Plank* The other, which is more properly fu ring, is to rip off the first Planks, and p other Timbers upon the first, and th the Planks upon those Timbers, which to make her bear a better Sail, for whe a Ship is too narrow, and the Bearing e ther not laid out enough, or too lo they must make her broader, and lay h Bearing higher They commonly fu two or three Strakes under Water, and much above, according as the Ship r quires, more or less

Futtocks This Word more proper should be *Foot-Hooks*, but is ever pronounc *Futtocks*, which are those compassing Ti bers that give the Breadth and Bearing the Ship, and are scarf'd to the Groun Timbers And because no Timbers th compass can be found long enough to up through all the Side of the Ship, the compassing Timbers are scarf'd into t others, and those next the Keel are call the *Lower Ground-Futtocks*, and the othe the *Upper Futtocks*

G.

TO *Gage*, is to measure how much Cask contains To gage a Ship, to measure how much Water she dra

w b

when a float; and this is done by sticking a Nail into a Pike or Pole, which being put down by the Rudder, till the Nail catch hold under it, shows how much is under Water

A Gale, signifies the Wind, as, an easy or a lorm Gale, is little Wind, a fresh, a stiff, and a strong Gale, much Wind. Sometimes it happens that two Ships being at a small Distance from one another, the one shall be becalm'd, and the other have a little Wind, and then they say, she that has the Wind does gale away from the other

Gallery, is that beautifying Frame that is made upon the Stern of a Ship, without Board, into which there is a Passage out of the Great Cabbin, and are only for Show and Pleasure There are those on the Sides of the Stern which are of Use, as serving for necessary Houses

The Garboard, is the first Plank that is brought on the outside of the Ship, next the Keel.

The Garboard-Strake; is the first Strake, that is, the'first Seam next to the Keel, being the most dangerous Place in all the Ship to spring a-Leak, because it is almost impossible to come at it within Board

The Garland, is a Rope about the Main-Mast-Head, otherwise call'd the *Collar*, and serves to save the Shrowds from galling.

The Garnet; is a Tackle wherewith they hoise in all Casks and Goods, if they be not too heavy, as Ordnance, or the like

Gest-Rope, is a Rope belonging to th Boat, to keep her from sheering, whe she is tow'd after the Ship by the Boat Rope

Gift-Rope, is the same as Boat-Rope serving to tow the Boat after the Ship

Girding Vide *Trusses*

Girt When the Cable is so taug't that, upon the turning of the Tide, th Ship cannot go over it with her Stern-Post then she lies a-cross the Tye, and they say, she is Girt which ceases immediately, if the Cable be veer'd out slack

Glasses, are the Hour, Four Hour, and Minute Glasses, us'd at Sea, and they commonly call so many Hours, so many Glasses

Gone out a-Head, imports, that one Ship in sailing has pass'd before the Head of the other

Goreing A Sail is cut goreing, when it comes sloping by Degrees, and is broader at the Clew than at the Earing, as all Top-Sails and Topgallant-Sails are

Goosewing; is the Mizzen-Sail, boom'd out, to give the Ship more Way before a Wind

Grapnels, are in the Nature of Anchors for Gallies or Boats to ride by, but have four Flooks, and never a Stock They are also us'd in Men of War to fling into another Ship, and take hold of the Gratings, Rails, Gun-Wales, *&c* with a Chain made fast to them, to lash the Ships together. There are other small

Grap-

Grapnels with three Hooks, but not broad like Flooks, with which they uſe to ſweep for Hawſes or ſmall Cables.

Gratings, are ſmall Ledges laid over a-croſs one another, like a Portcullis, or a Priſon-Gate, and ſerve to let down light, and give Air betwixt the Decks.

To Grave, is to bring a Ship to lie dry aground, and then burn off all the old Filth and Stuff with Reed, Broom, or the like, and ſo lay on new, the beſt of which is Train-Oil, Rozen and Brimſtone, boil'd together.

The Gripe, is the Compaſs and Sharp-neſs of the Stem under Water, eſpecially towards the lower Part.

To Gripe. They ſay, a Ship gripes, when ſhe is apt, contrary to the Helm, to run her Head more to the Wind than ſhe ſhould.

Ground, and *Grounding*. When a Ship is purpoſely brought to be trimm'd on the Ground, it is call'd Grounding, but when they are drove on by Streſs of Wea-ther or other Accident, they call it, run-ning or ſtriking aground. When they go a little Way, and come to an Anchor again, they call it, breaking Ground.

Ground-Timbers, are thoſe which are faſt laid over the Keel, and ſo bolted through the Keelſon into the Keel, and make the Floor of the Ship, and are therefore cal-led Ground-Timbers, becauſe the Ship reſts on them when ſhe lies aground.

Gudgins, are the Irons which are made fast to the Stern-Post, into which the Pintels of the Rudder are hang'd

To Gull When the Pin of a Block eats, or wears into the Sheever, it is call'd, Gulling So when a Yard rubs against the Mast, they say, *It will gull the Mast*

A Gulph, is any Parcel of the Sea which is large within, narrow at the Mouth, and has no other Way out but the same you come in

The Gunner, has Charge of all the Ordnance in the Ship, and all Things belonging to it, as Carriages, Spunges, Ladles and Rammers, Powder and Shot, and is to look to all that belongs to it in Time of Fight

The Gun-Wale, is that Piece of Timber which reaches on either Side the Ship from the Half-Deck to the Forecastle, being the uppermost Bend, as it were, which finishes the upper Walls of the Hull there and wherein they put the Stanshions which support the Waste-Trees, and this Name is given it, whether there be any Guns there or no The lower Part also of any Port, where the Ordnance lies, is call'd, the Gun-Wale

A Guy, is a Rope us'd to keep any weighty Thing that is hois'd into the Ship from swinging in too fast, when it is over the *Gun-Wale* There is another Rope called *a Guy*, which is fasten'd to the Fore-Mast at one End, and reev'd through a single Block, which is seaz'd to the Pen-

dant

dant of the Winding-Tackle, and so reev'd again through another, that is seaz'd to the Fore-Mast, somewhat lower than the first Part; and this is to hale forward the Pendant of the Winding-Tackle

H

TO *Hale*, is the same which others call pulling a Rope

Hale aboard the Tack, is, bring it down close unto the *Chess-Tree*

To Hail a Ship, is to call to her, to know whence she is, or whither bound, or the like, which is done in these Words, *Ho the Ship*, and the other answers, *Hoe*

Half-Deck. Vide *Deck*

Halliards, are the Ropes by which all the Yards are hois'd, except the Cross-Jack and Spritsail-Yard, which have none, as being ever flung, tho' in small Craft, they have Halliards to the Sprit-Sail

Hands, and *Handing* This last Word is us'd to deliver any thing about from one to another, and when they want more Men to do any Work, they call for more Hands, not more Men

A Handspeek, is a Wooden Leaver, us'd, instead of an Iron Crow, to traverse the Ordnance; and so to the Windlass in the Boat, or in the Ship, if they have Windlasses to heave the Anchor by.

The Harpings; is the Breadth of a Ship at the Bow. Some call the Ends of the

the Bends, which are fasten'd into the Stem, by this Name

Hatches; are, as it were, Trap Doors, which are in the Mid-Ship before the Main-Mast, open'd to let down Goods into the Hould, and therefore have a Shackle of Iron at each End to lift them by

Hatch-Way, is the Place perpendicularly over the Hatches

The Hawses, are those great round Holes under the Head, through which the Cables pass when the Ship is at Anchor *A bold Hawse*, is when it lies high from the Water

A Hawser, is a Three-strand Rope, or a little Cable, for that which is one Ship's Hawser, will be another's Cable The Use of them is to warp a Ship over a Bar The Main and Fore-Shrowds are made of Hawsers

The Head, is often taken for all the fore Part of the Ship Vide *Beak-Head*

The Head of the Anchor, is that Part in which the Eye is, through which the Ring passes

Head-Lines; are the uppermost Ropes of all Sails next the Yards, by which they are made fast to them

Head-Sails, are all those which belong to the Fore Mast, Spritsail, and Spritsail-Top Mast

Head-Sea After a great Storm, the Wind will sometimes suddenly alter six Points or more, but the Sea will go the same

same Way it did for some Hours, then if the Ship go with this Wind against the Sea, she will meet this Sea right a-Head, and therefore it is call'd, a *Head-Sea* In Head-Seas, all short Ships are bad Sailors

To Heave and Set, is when the Ship falls and rises with the Waves at Anchor

To Heave at the Capstain; is to work at or turn it about with the Bars, as is done to weigh Anchor, or bring any very weighty Thing aboard.

To Heave a Thing away; is to throw it away

To Heave over Board, to throw out of the Ship

The Heel, of the Main, Fore, and Mizen-Masts, is only that Part which is par'd away a little slanting, on the aftward Side of the Foot of the Mast, like a Heel, to give it Leave to be stay'd aftward on; but the Heels of the Top-Masts are Squares, and in them they put the Fidd of the Top-Mast

To Heel, is for the Ship to lie down on a Side, whether afloat or aground.

Height of the Sun, is its Meridian Elevation above the Horizon

The Helm, is that Piece of Timber which the Steersman holds in his Hand to steer and govern the Rudder, to which Purpose, one End of it is made fast to the Head of the Rudder, that it may be taken off This it is that directs and governs the Ship's Way.

To Hitch, is to catch any Thing with a Rope, or with a Hook.

The Hold Vid *Howld*

To hold off, is, when they heave the Cable at the Capstain. if it be very stiff and great, or have lain in a slimy owzi Ground, it surges and slips back, unless that Part which is heav'd in be still hal'd away hard from the Capstain, to keep the Cable close and hard to the Capstain Whelps If it be a small Cable, Men may do it with their Hands, but if great then either they hold off with Nippers, or else, as in all great Ships, they bring it to the Jeer-Capstain, and this is call'd *Holding off*

Hony-Comb'd, is when a Gun is full of small Holes within, either through a Fault in the Casting, or otherwise

The Hooks, are all those forked Timbers which are plac'd upright on the Keel both in the Rake and Run of the Ship They give the Narrowing and Breadthing of the Ship in these Parts, and are bolted into the Keel

A Horse, is a Rope made fast to one of the Fore-Mast-Shrowds, with a Dead Man's-Eye at the End of it, through which is reev'd the Pendant of the Spritsail Sheats; and is for no other Use but to keep the Spritsail-Sheats clear off the Flooks of the Anchor When a Man heaves the Head of the Shrowds, there is a Rope made fast to the Shrowds for him to lean against, for Fear of falling into

into the Sea, which is call'd, *a Horse* There is alſo a Rope to ſet taught the Shrowds, with Wale-Knots, one End made faſt to the Shrowds, to the other the Lanniers are brought; and ſo with a Hand-Speek turning it, they ſet taught the Halliards, and this bears the ſame Name of *a Horſe* Beſides, thoſe ſmall Ropes which are ſeaz'd to the middle of the Top-Maſt and Topgallant Stayes with a Block, wherein are reev'd the Topſail and Topgallant-Bowlings, are call'd Horſes

Hoſpital-Ships, are Veſſels fitted with Beds and other Conveniencies, as Surgeons, and all neceſſary Drugs, *&c* for the Sick and Wounded Men, that they may not encumber the Men of War.

The Howld All the Room between the Keelſon, and the firſt or lower Deck, is call'd the Hold, or Howld, and there all the Victuals, Stores and Goods, are lay'd; but it is divided into ſeveral Rooms with Bulk-Heads, as, the Steward's Room, the Powder Room, the Boatſwain's Room, *&c.*

The Hownds, are the Holes in the Cheeks, which are faſten'd to the Head of the Maſts, wherein the Ties run, to hoiſe the Yards The Top-Maſts have but one Hole aloft in the Head of the Maſt, becauſe they have but ſingle Ties; and this is alſo call'd *the Hownds*

Howſeing-in, is when a Ship, after ſhe is paſs'd the Breadth of her Bearing, is brought in narrow to her upper Works

A Hoy;

A Hoy; is a ſmall Bark, that ſails no with Croſs-Yards, but with Sails in th Form of Mizzen-Sails, and will ſail near er the Wind than any can do with Croſs Sails

To Hoyſe, is to hale any thing into th Ship with a Tackle or dead Rope, or g up a Yard, or the like

The Hull, is the Body or Bulk of th Ship without Maſts, Yards, Ropes, o Sails

Hulling; is when a Ship at Sea has ta ken in all her Sails, either in calm Wea ther or in a Storm

A Hullock, is a ſmall Part of a Sai which is loos'd and left open in a grea Storm, when we dare not have any mor out, and is only us'd in the Mizzen-Sai when we would keep the Ship's-Head t the Sea, with a little Sail, making all up excepting a little at the Mizzen-Yard Arm Elſe, when a Ship will not Wea ther-coile, to lay her Head the other way they looſe a Hullock of the Fore Sail, and changing the Helm to the Weather ſide the Ship will fall off, and lay her Hea where her Stern lay before

I

THE *Jeer*, is a Piece of a Hawſe made faſt to the Main and Fore Yards, cloſe to the Ties of great Ship for ſmall ones do not uſe it, and ſo it i reev'd through a Block which is ſeaz' clof close to the Top, and so comes down and is reev'd through another Block at the Bottom of the Mast, close by the Deck Great Ships have one on the one, and another on the other Side of the Ties The Use of this Rope is to help hoise up the Yard, but the chiefest is to succour the Ties, and to hold the Yard from falling down if the Ties should break

The Jeer-Capstan, has its Name from the Jeer, which is ever brought to this Capstan to be heav'd at by It stands in the Waste in the Hatch-way, and serves for many other Uses, as to heave upon the Viol, or hold off the Cable from the Main-Capstain Vide *Capstain*

Indraught, is a Place where the Sea runs in

Joyner Great Ships carry a Joyner to wainscot and adorn them

Iron Sick A Ship or Boat is said to be *Iron Sick*, when the Bolts, Speeks, or Nails, are so eaten away with the Rust or Salt-Water, that they stand hollow in the Planks, and the Vessel takes in Water by them, for which Reason they put Lead over all the Bolts-Heads under Water

A Junk, is any Piece of a Cable that is cut off, and such they hang for Fenders on the Ship's Sides.

A Jury-Mast, is either a spare Mast, or the Main or Fore-Yard, set up in the Place of the Main or Fore-Mast, when either of them is lost, either in Fight or bad Weather, and so fit a Yard, Sails and other

other Neceſſaries, to it, to make a Shi[ft] with it to ſteer the Ship, and get her in[to] Harbour

K

TO *Keckle*, or *Keckling*, is the twiſtin[g] of a ſmall Rope round the Cab[le] or the Bolt-Rope, when they fear the o[ne] ſhould gall in the Hawſe, and the oth[er] againſt the Quarter of the Ship, and th[at] ſaves them, which in all other Ropes [is] call'd Serving, and only in theſe two Kec[k]ling

A Kedger Vide *Anchor*

To Kedge, or *Kedging* In bringing [a] Ship up or down a narrow River, wh[en] the Wind is contrary to the Tide, th[ey] ſet the Fore-Sail, or Foretop-Sail a[nd] Mizzen, and ſo let her drive with t[he] Tide The Sails are to flat her about, [if] ſhe comes too near the Shore They a[lso] carry out an Anchor in the Head of t[he] Boat, with a Hawſer that comes from t[he] Ship, which Anchor, if the Ship com[es] too near the Shore, they let fall in t[he] Stream, and ſo wind her Head about [by] it, then weigh the Anchor again wh[en] ſhe is about, which is call'd *Kedging*, a[nd] from this Uſe, the Anchor a *Kedger*

The Keel, is the firſt Timber that [is] laid of a Ship, being the ſharp Botto[m] and, as it were, the Foundation of all [the] reſt, and ſo much is the *Kneel* as lies [in a] ſtrait Line betwixt Head and Stern, [...]

St[...]

Stem being scarf'd in at the one End, and the Stern-Post let in at the other All the Ground-Timbers, and Hooks fore and aft are bolted to it, and on them all the upper Works rais'd

A Rank-Keel, is a deep one, which is good to keep a Ship from rowling

A Showle-Keel, is that which lies not deep in the Water, and therefore the Ship is apt to rowl

A False Keel Vide *False*

The Keel-Rope, is one that runs along the Ship upon the Keel, within the Limbers of the Ground-Timbers, one End coming out before, and the other abaft The Use of it is to clear the Limber-Holes when they are stock'd with Ballast, or any thing else, so as the Water that lies betwixt the Timbers cannot come to the Well of the Pump

A Kenk When a Rope that should run smooth in a Block has got a little Turn, so that it comes double, they call it, a Kenk The same in the Cable, if it runs out doubling

A Ketch, is a small Vessel, such as come up to *Billingsgate* with Oysters, or the like

Kevels; are small Pieces of Timber nail'd on the inside of the Ship, to which they belay the Sheats and Tacks

A Knave Line; is a Rope fasten'd on the one End to the Chess-Trees, under the Main or Fore-Top, and so coming down by the Ties to the Ram-Head; to which

is

is seaz'd a small Piece of Billet, about two Foot long, with a Hole in the End of it, in which this Line is reev'd, and so brought to the Ship's Side, and hal'd up taught to the Rails The Use of it is to keep the Ties and Halliards from turning about one another when they are new; for when well stretch'd, there is no need of it

A Kneck, is the twisting together of a Rope that is not well quoil'd

Knees, are the crooked Timbers, so call'd, because they represent a Man's Knee bent, and serve to bind the Beams and Futtocks together, being bolted into them both

Kneetles, are two Rope Yarns twisted together, with a Knot at each End, to seaze a Rope or Block, or the like

A Knight, is a Piece of Timber in which are four Sheevers, three for the Halliards, and one for the Top-Rope, to run in when hoys'd, and has commonly the Figure of some Head carv'd on it, by which it is easily known There are two of these, the *Fore-Knight*, standing abaft the Fore-Mast, and the *Main-Knight* aft the Main-Mast, both fast bolted to the Beams

Knittlidge Vide *Ballast*

Knots That call'd a Bowling Knot, so made, that it will not slip nor slide The other a Wale-Knot, is a round Knob made with three Strands of a Rope, so that it cannot slip neither.

L

TO *Labour* A Ship is said to Labour in the Sea, when she rowls and tumbles very much, either a-Hull, or under Sail, or at an Anchor

To Lace, or *Lacing*, is the same as on Land, for they Lace on the Bonnet to the Sail, and the Drabler to the Bonnet, &c

Ladders There are three belonging to a Ship, the *Entring-Ladder* at the Waste, and the Ladder of Ropes which hangs out of the Gallery Vide *Entring-Ladder* The third is at the Beak-Head, to get up the Boltsprit by

To Lade, is to fill a Ship with Goods &c which is call'd *Lading* They also call it Lading of great Guns, which is, to charge them, and to lade the Water out of the Boat, or the like, is to throw it out

A Ladle, is like a Scoop at the End of a Pole, to put the Powder into a Gun, when they take it out of the Budge-Barrel

Land-Fall If they say, they shall see Land such a Day, and it happens accordingly, they say, they have a good Land Fall If they are mistaken, they say, they made a bad Land-Fall

Land Lock'd Roads or Harbours which are so encompass'd with Land, that the Sea cannot beat in to wrong a Ship, are said to be *Land-Lock'd*

Land-to, is just so far at Sea as they can see the Land

A Land-Turn; is a Wind blowing regularly off from the Land by Night, as the Brieze does off the Sea by Day

The Land is shut in, signifies, that it is hid from Sight by some other Land

Langrel, is a Shot which goes in with a Shackle to be shorten'd when put into the Piece, and to fly out at length when discharg'd, with a half Bullet at either End, good near-hand for cutting down of Masts, Yards, Ropes and Sails, and to destroy Men

Lanniers; are small Ropes, reev'd into the Dead-Men's-Eyes of all the Shrowds and Chains, the Use of them being to slacken or set taught the Shrowds Also the Stays belonging to the Masts are set taught by Lanniers. And the Rope which makes fast the Stopper of the Halliards to the Halliards, is call'd a *Lannier*

Larboard, is the Left Side of the Ship as a Man stands in her with his Face forward.

Large When a Ship goes neither by a Wind, nor before it, but betwixt both it is call'd, a Large Wind

To Lash, is to bind up any thing to the Ship's Sides, or Masts or the like

Lashers; are properly those Ropes which bind fast together the Tackles and Breechings of the Guns when they are hal'd within Board

Laskets Vide *Latchets*

Lasking A Ship is said to go Lasking, hen she neither goes by nor before a Vind

Latchets; are small Lines sown into the onnet and Drabler, like Loops, wherewith they lace the Bonnet to the Course, d the Drabler to the Bonnet, putting em into the Eyelet-Holes, and lacing em over one another.

Launch, signifies to put out; as to aunch a Ship, is to put her out of the ock into the Water, and so in other ases But us'd also in another Sense, as hen they have hoys'd up a Yard high ough, or the Top-Mast, they cry, *unch hoa*; that is, hoyse no more, and stowing the Hould, they say, *Launch* , or *Launch forward*, when they would ave any Goods brought forward or aftard So in pumping, when the Pump cks, they cry, *Launch hoa*, that is, pump o more

To Lay the Land. When they have sail'd ut of Sight of Land, they say, they have aid the Land

A Leak A Ship is said to Leak, when e makes more Water than ordinary; or there is none so tight but she may ake some

Ledges, are those small Pieces of Timer which come athwart Ships from the Waste-Trees to the Roof-Trees, to bear p the Nettings

Lee The *Lee* is generally that Side which is opposite to the Wind, as the Lee-

Lee-Shore, is that the Wind blows on To be under the Lee of the Shore, is t be cloſe under the Weather-Shore Leeward Ship, is one that is not faſt b a Wind to make her Way ſo good as ſh might To come by the Lee, or lay Ship by the Lee, is to bring her ſo th all her Sails may lie againſt the Maſts an Shrowds flat, and the Wind to com right on her Broad-ſide, ſo that ſhe wi make little or no Way

The Lee-Fang, is a Rope reev'd into th Creengles of the Courſes, when the would hale in the Bottom of the Sail, t lace on the Bonnet In a ſtrong G they ſerve alſo to take in the Sail

The Lee-Latch When he who con would bid the Man at Helm to look th the Ship does not go to Leeward of h Courſe, he bids him have a Care of th *Lee-Latch*

Lee ſeel, is the tumbling of a Ship t Leeward, when the Water forſakes h on that Side

The Leetch, is the outward Side Skirt of the Sail, from the Earing to th Clew, the middle Part whereof is mo eſpecially the *Leetch*

Leetch-Lines, are ſmall Lines ma faſt to the Leetch of the Topſails, an no others, and reev'd into a Block at th Yard, cloſe by the Topſail-Ties, th Uſe whereof is, when they take in th Topſails, to hale in the Leetch of th Sail

Legs

Legg's, are small Ropes, call'd the Leggs of the Martnet, put through the Bolt-Rop s of the Main and Fore-Sail, near a oot in Length, and being splic'd into hemselves at either End, they have a lit-e Eye, into which the Martnets are made ast, with two Hitches, and the End seaz'd the standing Part of the Martnets

Let fall, is the Phrase generally us'd or putting out of any Sails, when the ards are aloft, but not to the Top-Sails, or which the proper Term is, *Heave out*; or for the Mizzen, for which the Term , *Set the Mizzen* *Let fall the Anchor*, is, it go down into the Sea

Let fly the Sheat; is, let it run out vio-ntly, as far as it can go

The Lifts, are Ropes belonging to the rd-Arms of all the Yards, and only ve to top the Yard-Arms, that is, to ke them hang higher or lower, as y please, but the Topsail-Lifts serve Sheats to the Topgallant-Yards The ing of them is call d, Topping the ts

Lumbers or *Lumber-Holes*, are little square les cut in the Bottom of all the ound-Timbers and Hooks, next to the el, the Use whe eof is to let the Wa-r pass to the Well of the Pump

Linspins, are only us'd about the Trucks the Carriages, to keep on the Trucks on the Axletree, being little Iron Pins, e those that keep on Coach-Wheels.

M

Lockers, are little Boxes like Cupboards some by the Guns to lay Shot in, and in other Places for other Uses

A Log-Line, or, as some call it, a *Minute-Line*, is a small Line, with a little Piece of Board at the End of it, and on it a Bit of Lead, to keep it Edge-long in the Water This being cast into the Sea, and the Line heav'd out after it for a Minute, by a Minute-Glass, shews how many Fathom the Ship runs in that Minute, and by it they make a Judgment how many Leagues she runs in a Watch or four Hours

The Long-Boat, is the strongest and biggest of the Boats belonging to a Ship, and serves to carry all weighty Things to her, to land Men upon Occasion, to weigh the Anchor, and many other Uses

The Loof, is that Part aloft of the Ship which lies just before the Chess-Trees, as far as the Bulk-Head of the Castle, whence the Guns lying there are call'd, Loof-Pieces

Loof-up A Term us'd in Conding, to have the Man at the Helm keep the Ship nearer the Wind To Loof into a Harbour, is to keep close to the Wind, and so get in keep your Loof is, keep close to the Wind To spring ones Loof, is when the Ship is going large, to clap close by a Wind

A Loof-Hook, is a Tackle with two Hooks, one to hitch into a Creengle of the Main and Fore-Sail, which Creengle is in the Bolt-Rope of the Leetch of the Sail, not far above the Clew; and the other to hitch into a Strop, which is plac'd into the Chess-Tree, and so to bowse down the Sail The Use of it, to succour the Tackle in a great Gale.

A Loom-Gale Vide *Gale*

To Loom When they say, a Ship looms a great Sail, it signifies, she seems to be a large Ship, and she looms but small, is, she shews little; so that *Looming* is the Appearance or the Perspective they have of a Ship

A Lust When a Ship heels a little to either Side, they say, she has a Lust that Way

To lie under the Sea, signifies, that the Ship lies a-Hull, with her Helm made fast a Lee, so as the Sea breaks upon her Bow and Broad-side

M

TO *Man a Ship*, is to give her the due Complement of Men.

Man the Capstain, is, put Men to work at the Capstain. And so in other Cases

A Man of War, is always meant of Ships for Fight

The Manger, is a Place, made with Planks fasten'd on the Deck, a Foot and half high, right under the Hawse, sometimes in a Triangle; the Use whereof is to receive the Water that comes in at the Hawses, when the Ship rides at Anchor in great

 Stresses,

Streſſes, that then Water may not run on upon the Decks, and ſo into the Hould

Marlin, is a ſmall Line, made of untwiſted Hemp, to be more pliant, and is alſo Tarr'd. The Uſe of it, to ſeaze the Ends of Ropes from farſing out, and for other Uſes

Marlin-Speek; is a ſmall Iron Speek made on purpoſe for the ſplicing together of ſmall Ropes, and to open the Bolt-Ropes when they ſew in the Sail

Martnets, are ſmall Lines, faſten'd to the Legs, on the Leetch of the Sail

The Maſter, has the whole Charge of ſailing the Ship abroad at Sea, and accordingly commands all next to the Captain and Lieutenant in Men of War, but is Chief in Merchants, and therefore vulgarly call'd Captain, tho' it be not his Due.

Maſts; are thoſe Trees ſtanding upright in Ships, which carry the Yards Tops, and Rigging Great Ships have three Maſts, the Fore-Maſt, next the Head, the Main-Maſt, in the Middle and the Mizzen-Maſt, next the Stern Each of theſe has a Top-Maſt on its Head and the Fore and Main Top-Maſts their Topgallant-Maſts over them

Mats; are broad Clouts wove with Sinnet and Thrums together, or without Thrums; us'd to ſave Things from gauling

Metal, generally ſignifies the Quantity, not the Quality of it. To diſpert the Metal

Metal. Vide *Dispert*. The Piece is laid under Metal, signifies, that her Mouth is lower than her Breech. Over Metal, is the contrary. Right with her Metal, is, when the Piece lies point-blank.

Minute-Line. Vide *Log-Line*.

The Mizzen, absolutely spoken, signifies the Sail, not the Mast.

Mizzen-Mast. Vide *Mast*.

Mizzen Sail. Vide *Sail*.

Mizzen-Stay. Vide *Stay*.

Mizzen-Top-Mast. Vide *Top-Mast*.

Mizzen-Yard. Vide *Yard*.

To Moor, or *Mooring*. This is done several Ways. First, *To Moor a-Cross*, or *thwart*, is to lay one Anchor on one Side of a River, and another on the other, right against it, so as both Cables may bear together, either for Ebb or Flood. *To Moor alongst*, is to lay one Anchor right in the Middle of the Stream on a-Head, and the other a-Stern. The Third, is *Mooring Water-Shot*, that is, quartering between both, for it is neither a-Cross nor alongst the Tide. A Ship is not said to Moor with less than two Anchors aground.

To Mount a Gun, is either to put it into the Carriage, or else, when in the Carriage, to raise the Mouth higher.

Munk-Seam; is a Way of sewing the Canvas of the Sails together, the Edge of the one over the Edge of the other, and so sown on both Sides, which is the strongest Way.

Murderers, are ſmall Pieces with Chambers, charg'd with Murdering-Shot to ſcour the Decks

N

NEale to That is, deep Water cloſe to the Shore, without any Showling.

Neap-Tide, is oppoſite to the Spring-Tide, and happens in the midſt of the ſecond and laſt Quarter of the Moon; and there are as many Days allow'd for the Neap or Falling of the Tides, as for the Spring or Riſing of them In Neap-Tides, the Water is never ſo high nor ſo low as in the Spring-Tides, nor do they run ſo ſwift As the Higheſt of the Spring is three Days after the Full or Change of the Moon, ſo the Loweſt of the Neap is four Days before the Full or Change, and that is call'd, the *Dead-Neap*. When a Ship has not Water enough to bring her off the Ground or Dock, they ſay, ſhe is Beneap'd

The Needle, is the Iron Wire made faſt to the Fly of the Compaſs, and which gives Motion to it, as being touch'd with a Loadſtone

Nettings, are thoſe ſmall Ropes which are ſeaz'd together with Rope-Yarns, in the Form of a Net, with Maſhes, and for the moſt Part only us'd in the Waſte

Netting Sails, are the Sails they lay upon the Nettings

Nippers, are small Ropes, a Faddom and half or two Faddom long, with a little Truck at one End, or only a Wale Knot, the Use whereof is to hold off the Cable from the Main-Capstain or the Jeer-Capstain, when they cannot do it with their Hands.

No Near, is a Term in Conding, to bid the Man at the Helm go more large, or before the Wind.

The Nut of the Anchor. Vide *Anchor*.

O

TO *Observe*, or *take an Observation*, is to take the Height of the Sun or Star with any Instrument, to find the Latitude the Ship is in.

Ockham, is nothing but old Ropes untwisted and pull'd out into loose Flax again. New Toe and Flax, us'd in the same Manner, is also call'd, White Ockham. The Use of them is to drive into the Seams of the Planks, to keep out the Water, and to make small Lines for common Uses.

The Offing. That is, the Part out in the open Sea from the Shore.

Offward. When a Ship is ashore, and heels to the Waterward, they say, she heels to the Offward; or if her Stern lie towards the Sea, they say, it lies to the Offward.

Orlop, is the same as Deck, only if a Ship have three Decks they never call the uppermost of them an Orlop, but the other two are more properly call'd Orlops than Decks. Vide *Deck*.

To Overhale, is, when a Rope is hal'd too stiff or taught, to hale it the contrary Way, and make it slacker.

Over-raking, is when the Sea over-washes a Ship from Stem to Stern as she rides at Anchor, by reason of her over-beating her self into a Head-Sea.

Overset, is turn'd topsie-turvy, or over-turn'd at Sea. Also the turning over of a Cable or small Rope that is quoil'd up, is call'd Oversetting.

Overthrown, is a Ship that, being brought to be trimm'd aground, falls over on a Side.

The Out-licker, is a small Piece of Timber, two or three Yards long, made fast to the Top of the Poop, and standing out-right a-Stern, at the outwardmost End whereof is a Hole, into which the standing Part of the Sheat is made fast, and being reev'd through the Block of the Sheet, is reev'd again through another Block, which is seaz'd to this Piece of Tim[illegible], near the End, and so the Use [illegible] to hale down the Mizzen-Sheat [illegible]. This is us'd in few Ships, and [illegible] small ones.

Owze, is soft, slimy, muddy Ground, very bad for Anchoring, but good to lay a Ship aground on.

P

THE *Pallet*, is a Room in the Hould sever'd from the rest, in which a few Pigs of Lead, or such weighty Matter, being stow'd, the Ship may be sufficiently Ballasted, with the Loss of little Room in her Hould.

A Parbuncle, is a Rope us'd in the Nature of a Pair of Slings, to hoise in the Cask.

To Parcel, or *Parcelling*, is to take a little Canvas about the Breadth of a Hand, and lay it over a Seam which is first caulk'd; then heat a little Pitch and Tar very hot, and pour it over the Canvas.

Parrels, are those Things made of Trucks, and Ribs and Ropes, which go about the Mast, and are at both Ends made fast to the Mast, so contriv'd with the Trucks and Ribs, that the Yard may slide up easily.

The Partners, are the Timbers that are bolted to the Beams, and compass the Shoot in the Mast at the Deck, being the Strength, and keep up the Mast steady in the Step. There are also Partners in the second Deck, that it may not rowl out the Ship's Sides, but the Mizzen has only one Pair of Partners.

A Passarado, or more properly, a *Nepasmua-Rope*, is any Rope wherewith they hale down the Sheat-Blocks of the Main and Fore Sails, when they are hal'd aft the Clew of the Main Sail, to the Cub-bridge-Head of the Main-Mast, and the Clew of the Fore-Sail to the Cat-Head, which is done when the Ship goes large

The Pawl, is a little Piece of Iron bolted to one End of the Beams or the Deck, close to the Capstain, but so easily, that it has Leave to turn about, and against this the Whelps of the Capstain bear, when they would have it held from turning back again

Pawl the Capstain, is, turn it up to the Pawl, that it may hold it from turning back

Pawnches; are Mats made of Sinnet, fasten'd to the Main and Fore-Yards, to save them from gauling

To Pay, is to lay hot Pitch upon a Seam, after caulking of it It is also call'd Paying, when, after a Ship is grav'd, they lay on the Stuff, whatever it be, Rozen and Brimstone, and Oil, or the like They also say, a Ship is Pay'd, when she is to tack, and all her Sails are a-Back-Stays, that is, flat against the Shrowds and Masts

A-Peek; as, to heave a-Peek, is to bring the Hawse of the Ship right over the Anchor, so that the Cable is then right perpendicular betwixt them

To Ride a-Peek; is to have the Main Yard and Fore-Yard hois'd up, and one End brought up close to the Shrowds, up and down the contrary Ways, so that the two Yards make a *St. Andrew*'s Cross.

The

The Peek, is the Room in the Ship's Hould, from the Bits forward to the Stem

Peek the Mizzen, is, put the Yard right up and down by the Mast

Pendant, is a short Rope, made fast at one End either to the Head of the Mast or to the Yard, or to the Clew of the Sail, and has at the other End a Block with a Sheever, to reeve some running Rope into it All the Yard Arms, except the Mizzen, have Pendants, into which the Braces are reev'd Pendants are also those Colours which are hung out on the Yard-Arms, or from the Head of a Mast, for a Shew, and to beautify the Ship

The Pillow, is the Timber on which the Boltsprit rests, at the coming out of the Hull of the Ship aloft by the Stem

A Pilot, is one who conducts Ships into Roads and Harbours, and over Bars and Sands, and through dangerous Channels, or such-like Places

Pintels; are small Iron Pins made fast to the Rudder, by which the Rudder hangs to the Stern-Post

Pitching, is not only laying on Pitch, which is properly call'd Paying, but is the placing the Step of the Mast And if a Ship falls much into a Sea, they say, she Pitches, and if she endangers her Masts by it, they say, she will pitch her Masts by the Board.

Plate the Cable; is the same as serve the Cable. Vide *Serve*

Plats, are flat Ropes, made of Rope-Yarn, woven one over another, and are to save the Cable in the Hawse from gauling

A Plot, is the same as a Sea-Card Vide *Card*

A Point The Sharpness of any Head-Land is call'd, the Point of Land The Compass is also divided into 32 Points, representing so many Winds

The Poop, is the uppermost Part a Stern of the Ship's Hull, being the Deck over that which is commonly call'd, the Master's-Cabbin

Ports, are the Places out of which the Guns are put through the Ship's Sides

To Port, is a Word us'd in Conding the Ship, when she sails right before a Wind and signifies to put the Helm to the Larboard Side

Pouches, are small Bulk-Heads made in the Hould, either athwart or alongst Ships, which serve either to keep Goods that will not stow well, or the Ballast from shifting

Powder There are two Sorts of it, the one call'd Serpentine, which is in Dust without corning, never us d at Sea, the other Corn-Powder, whereof there are several Sorts, but those us'd at Sea are only two, the Cannon Powder, which is large Corn, and not very strong, and Musket Powder, fine, and very strong The Ingredients for making of Powder, are Saltpetre, which gives the Force, Brimstone and Charcoal.

The

The Powder-Room; is the Place in the ould where the Powder is kept

Preddy, is us'd among Sailors instead Ready

A Preventure Rope, is a little Rope feaz'd er a cross the Ties, close at the Ram-ad, that if one Part of the Ties should eak, the other should not run through e Ram-Head, to endanger the Yard

Priming, is putting the Powder to the ouch-hole of any Piece for firing It also the Ground or first Colour, laid for ers to come over in painting a Ship.

A Priming-Horn, is that in which the nner keeps Powder for priming of the ns

A Priming-Iron, is a small sharp Iron ich they thrust in at the Touch-hole a Gun, to make Way through the Car-idge for the Priming-Powder to meet th the Charge

A Proviso; is a Hawser carry'd ashore, en a Ship has one Anchor out, and en she is said to be moor'd with her ad to the Shore

The Prow, is the foremost Part of the ip aloft, and not below between Decks, in Hould

The Prow-Pieces, are those which lie a-before

Puddings, are Ropes nail'd round to the rd-Arms of the Main and Fore-Yards, se to the End, and so in three or four, more Distances, one from another, up-each Yard-Arm. The Use of them, is to to ſave the Robbins from gauling aſund upon the Yards, when they hale home t Topſail-Sheats So the ſerving of t Ring of the Anchor with Ropes, ſave the Clinch of the Cable from ga ing againſt the Iron, is call'd, the Pu ding of the Anchor

Pullies, are ſmall Blocks, with one two Sheevers in them, but great ones not call'd Pullies

Pumps There are three Sorts of th us'd in Ships. The firſt and common are ordinary Pumps, ſuch as are us'd ſhore, which ſtand by the Main M The next is a Bar-Pump, not us'd *Engliſh* Ships, but *Flemmings* have th in their Sides, and are call'd by the Na of Bildge-Pumps, becauſe they have bro long Floats, which hold much Bild Water This Pump delivers more Wa than the other, and is not ſo laborious work at The third and laſt is the Cha Pump, which delivers moſt Water, a with moſt Eaſe, and ſooneſt mended any thing chance to give Way Th are alſo ſmall Pumps which they put to the Bung of a Cask, to pump out W ter or any Liquor

The Pump-Brake, is the Handle th pump with at the ordinary ſort of Pum

The Pump-Can, is the Can they dr Water in to pour into the Pumps

The Pump Dale; is the Trough wher the Water runs along the Decks to t Skupper-Holes.

To Purchase, is to bring in, or gain upon a Rope they hale at So they say, the Capstain does Purchase apace, that is, brings in the Cable apace

Purser, is an Officer aboard a Ship, who is to receive the Quantity of Provisions, according to the Ship's Company, from the Victualler, for the Time the Ship is to be Victualled, and see it well stow'd. He is also to keep a List of all the Men.

Puttocks, are the small Shrowds, which go from the Shrowds of the Main, Fore and Mizzen Masts, to the Tops, and from the Top-Mast-Shrowds to the Top-Gallant; the Use of them being to go from the Shrowds into the Tops, because, when the Shrowds come near up to the Mast, they fall in so much, that the Men could not get into the Tops from them These Puttocks are from the Bottom Laz'd to a Staff, made fast there to the Shrowds, and above to a Plate of Iron, or to a Dead-Man's-Eye, to which the Lanniers of the Fore-Mast-Shrowds do come

Q

THE *Quarter*, is that Part of the Hull of the Ship, that reaches from the Steeridge to the Transome or Fashion-Piece

A fat Quarter; is a broad Quarter.

The Quarter-Deck; is the Deck over the Steeridge till it come to the Master's Cabbin Vide *Deck*. *Quar-*

Quartering; is when a Gun lies so, and may be so travers'd, that it will shoot on the same Line, or Point of the Compass as the Quarter bears When a Ship sails with Quarter-Winds, they say, she goes Quartering

The Quarter-Master, is an Officer who has Charge to rummage the Hould, to over-look the Steward, and see there be no Abuse or Waste committed, to look to the Loading of the Ship, and to Cond

Quarter-Watch, is when a Quarter of the Ship's Company watches, which is us'd in Harbour, when there is no Danger; for at other Times half the Company watches

Quarter Winds, are those that come over abaft the Main-Mast-Shrowds, just with the Quarter

A Quoyle, is a Rope laid up round, one Take over another Sometimes it is taken for a whole Rope quoyl'd, so that if half the Rope be cut away, they say, there is but half a Quoyle of that Rope

To Quoyle, is to lay the Takes of a Rope round over one another, so that they may run out smooth upon Occasion, without any Knecks; and also to lie handsomely in the Ship

Quoyns There are three Sorts of them us'd in a Ship, that is, the Quoyns the Gunners use under the Guns, to mount them higher or lower. They are broad, but thinner at one End than the other, being perfect broad Wedges, with a Handle ck at the thick End to draw them out or put them farther in, as Occasion requires Another Sort are call'd Cantick-Quoyns, being short, with three Edges, to put betwixt the Cask at the Bildge-Hoops, to keep the Cask steady from rowling and labouring one against another. The third are the standing Quoyns, made of Barrel-Boards, about four Fingers broad, and a fit Length to be driven a-cross betwixt the Buts, one End two or three Hoops from the thin Hoops of one But, and the other in the same Manner to the other, to keep the Chine of the But steady from jogging

R.

Rabbet of the Keel; is a hollowing away in the Keel for to let in the Planks to it

Rabbetting, is the letting in of the Planks to the Keel, hollow'd away to that Purpose in the Rake and Run, but not in the flat Floor

The Rake, is so much of the Ship's Hull as over-hangs both Ends of the Keel The Rake forward on is commonly more than a third, but less than half the Length of the Keel The Rake aftward is only for Beauty, and therefore but a fourth or fifth Part of her Rake forward

Ram-Head, is a great Block, with three Sheevers in it, in which are the Halliards, and at the Head of it into a Hole are reev'd

reev'd the Ties; and this Block only belongs to the Main and Fore Halliards

A Rammer, is a Staff with a roun
Piece of Wood at the End of it, som
what less than the Bore of the Gun it
to serve, and is to drive home the Ch-rg
in it

Ranges There are two of them, o
aloft upon the Forecastle, a little ab
the Fore-Mast, the other in the B
Head, before the Wouldings of the Bol
sprit. That in the Forecastle is a In
Piece of Timber, which goes over fro
the one Side to the other, and is the
fasten'd to the Timbers, and has tw
Knees about the Middle, on either Si
of the Fore-Mast, fasten'd to the Dec
and the Timber in which run the To
Sail-Sheats in a Sheever, and it has dive
Wooden Pins through it, to belay t
Ropes to. The other in the Beak-He
is in the same Form with the former

Ratling, is a Line, whereof they ma
the Steps by which they go up to t
Shrowds and the Puttocks, and so to t
Top-Mast-Shrowds, in great Ships, a
these Steps, which make the Shrowds l
Ladders, are call'd, the Ratlings of t
Shrowds

A Reach; is the Distance of any t
Points of Land, which bear in a rig
Line to one another, and is a Term m
commonly us'd in Rivers, as *Greenwi*
Reach, and the like

To Reeve; is no other in Respect to Ropes than putting them in, or passing them through, as they say, *Reeve the Tack through the Chess-Trees*, that is, pass it through, or, *Reeve the Halliards in the Knights and Ram-Heads*, that is, pass them through, and is generally understood of all Ropes that pass through Blocks, Dead-Mens-Eyes, Chess-Trees, or the like So when they would have a Rope pull'd out of the Block, they say, *Unreeve it*

Rends, are Cracks or Openings in the Planks, which they caulk to keep out the Water.

Ribs, are all those Timbers in general on which the Planks are laid, tho' they have particular Names, but are call'd Ribs from their Resemblance with those in a Man's Body. Also those little long Pieces, which are made with Holes under the Beak-Head, and belong to the Parrels of the Yards, are call'd, *the Ribs of the Parrels*.

To Ride A Ship Rides when her Anchors hold her fast, so that she does not drive away with the Tide or Wind, for tho' she sheer from one Side to the other, yet if her Anchors hold fast, and come not home, they say, she Rides.

To Ride a good Road, is to Ride where the Sea and Wind have much Power over the Ship, and strain her Cables very hard

To Ride a-cross; is to Ride with the Main-Yards and Fore-Yards hois'd up to the Hounds, and both Yard-Arms topp'd a-like

To

To Ride a-Peek, is to Ride with th Yards peek'd a-Peck, or else to Ride wi the Hawse just over the Anchor as whe a Ship is ready to sail

To Ride a Hawse-fall, is to Ride a gre Rode and Stress, signifying, that the W ter broke into the Hawses

To Ride thwart. is to Ride with th Ship's Side to the Tide, and then she n ver strains her Cables

To Ride betwixt Wind and Tide, is wh the Wind and Tide have equal Power, on one Way, and the other the contrary, that the Ship lies rowling with her Broa Side in the Trough of the Sea, when sh will rowl much, but not strain her Cable

Riders, are great Timbers, in the Hou or elsewhere, which do not properly b long to the Built of the Ship, but on bolted on upon the other Timbers, t strengthen them where they find the Shi weak

Rigging This Word comprehends a the Ropes that belong either to Masts o Yards, and they say, the Mast is Rigg and the Yard is Rigg'd, when they h v all the Ropes that belong to them

Right the Helm, is, keep it directly i the Middle of the Ship

Right the Yard, is, bring it to its prop Posture, when it has been out of it

Ring of the Anchor Vide *Anchor*.

Ring Bolts Vide *Bolts*

Rise the Tack, is as much as ease it or, as Landmen say, slacken it

The Risings, are those thick Planks that go fore and aft on both Sides under the Ends of the Beams and Timbers of the Second Deck, the Third Deck, and the Spirit and Quarter-Deck, whereon the Beams and Timbers of these Decks bear at both Ends by the Ship's Sides, but those thick Planks which in like manner bear up the lower Deck, are call'd *Lamps*

Rising Timbers, are the Hooks plac'd on the Keel, so call'd, because according to their rising by little and little, so the Rake and the Run of the Ship rise by Degrees from her flat Floor

A Road, is any Place where a Ship may ride near the Land, and yet not Land-lock'd for all Winds A good Road, is where there is good Ground for Anchor-hold, Showl-Water, and no great Sea-Gate coming in, however the Wind blows, the Land sheltering the one Side, and Sands, Rocks, or the like, breaking off the Sea on the other

A Wild Road, is where there is little Land on any Side, but all open to the Sea

A Roader, is any Ship that rides at an Anchor in a Road

Robbins, are little Lines reev'd into the Oylet-Holes of the Sail, under the Rope-Head, and serve to make fast the Sail to the Yard

The Roof-Trees, are the Timbers that go from the Half-Deck to the Forecastle, and serve to bear up the Gratings and Ledges where the Nettings are fasten'd, and are sup-

supported by Stanchions. That Piece o
Timber is also call'd a Roof-Tree, that
us'd upon Occasion, to be lay'd over th
Half-Deck, for Nettings, or any Sail, o
Pieces of Canvas to be laid upon it

Room, is large, broad and spacio
within Board

Ropes Generally all the Cordage b
longing to a Ship, is call'd by the Na
of Ropes, so a Cable is said to be a go
Rope, or a bad Rope, but in particul
there are some that have the Word Ro
added to their distinctive Appellatio
and are, *an Entring-Rope*, *a Bolt-Rope*,
Buoy-Rope, *a Guest-Rope*, *a Keel-Rope*, *a T*
Rope, *a Bucket-Rope*, *a Rudder-Rope*, *a P*
venture-Rope, and *a Brest-Rope* All whi
see in their Places

Rope-Yarns; are the Yarn of any Ro
untwisted, or more commonly of
Ends of worn Cables, and are for ma
Uses, as to serve small Ropes with, a
make Sinnet for Masts, or the like,
also *Knettles*, which are two of them t
sted together, and *Caburns* They are
so to wake up the Yard-Arms of the Sa

Rove and *Clinch* The Rove is the li
Iron Plate to which the Clinch-Nails
clinch'd And thus the Planks of Clinc
Boats are fasten'd together, which
of Work is call'd, *Rove* and *Clinch*

The Round-House, is the uppermost Ro
on the Stern of a Ship, and commonl
the Master's Cabbin.

Round

Round-in, is a Term us'd to the Main and Fore-Sail When the Wind larges upon them, they let rise the Main or Fore-tack and hale aft the Fore-Sheat to the Cat Head, and the Main-Sheat to the *Cubbridge-Head*, which they call, *Rounding aft*, or Rounding in the Sail

The Rowl, is the round Piece of Wood or Iron through which the Whip goes, being made to turn about, that it may carry over the Whip with more Ease from Side to Side

Rowse-in, is the Term us'd when a Cable and Hawser lies slack in the Water, and they would have it made taught; but this Word is not us'd in haling in of any other Rope

The Rudder, is that Piece of Timber which hangs at the Stern-Post of the Ship, on four, five, or six Irons, call'd Pintels, fitted for the Gudgins of the Stern-Post; and this is the Bridle that turns and winds the Ship any Way, for as this is turn'd, so the Ship's Head answers, and turns with it The putting on of the Rudder is call'd Hanging of it. The Part or Edge of it next the Stern-Post is call'd, the Inside, and the aftermost Part, the Rake of the Rudder

The Rudder-Rope; is a Rope or Strap reev'd into one Hole of the Rudder, near the Head and so likewise through the Stern-Post, and both Ends splic'd together, and serves to save the Rudder, if it chance to be beaten off, when the Ship sticks aground

Rudder-

Rudder-Irons; are the Cheeks of th Iron, whereof the Pintel is part, an these are fasten'd and nail'd round abou the Rake of the Rudder

To Rummidge, is to remove any Good or Luggage out of any Place betw Decks, but most commonly this Word us'd to remove and clear Things in th Ship's Hould, so that it may be we stow'd

The Run; is that Part of the Ship's Hu which is under Water, and comes thin ner and lanker away by Degrees, from th Floor Timber along to the Stern-Pos It is also call'd, *The Ship's Way aftward* o because, as she has either a good or ba Run, so the Water passes away swiftly o slowly alongst her, and the Ship mak more Way A Ship is said to have good Run, when it is long, and comes o handsomely by Degrees, and her Tac does not lie too low, which hinders th Water from coming swiftly and strong to the Rudder. The Run is of great Con sequence for the Ship's sailing, for if th Water come not swiftly to the Rudde she will not steer well; and the Ship th does not steer well, cannot sail we Merchant-Men do not generally give much Run as Men of War, because th Narrowing in of the Ships below los much Stowage

Rung-Heads; are the Heads or Ends the Rungs, which are made a little com passing, and do, as it were, lead or dire

t

he Sweep and Mould of the *Futtocks*, or in these Rungs, the Lines which give the Compass and Bearing of the Ship be-in The outward Ends of the Hooks, which are in the same manner compass-ing, are also call'd *Rung-Heads*, for the leeper, which is bolted in the other *ung Heads*, is also bolted into these

The Rungs, are the Ground-Timbers hat make the Floor of the Ship They e bolted into the Keel, and are strait, xcept at the Ends, where they begin to ompass a little

The Runner, is a Rope that is partly elonging to the Garnet and the two olt Tackles, that before, which comes the aftermost Shrowds of the Fore-last, and that Tackle abaft, which comes the foremost Shrowds of the Main-Mast It is reev'd in a single Block, hich is seaz'd to the End of the Pen-ant, and has at one End a Hook to hitch to any thing, and at the other End a ouble Block, in which is reev'd the Fall the Tackle, or the Garnet, which pur-hases more than the Tackle or Garnet ould do without it, and therefore this us'd to heavy Things. But for lighter, ey only use the Tackle with the Hook, hich is seaz'd to the standing Part of e Fall To over-hale the Runner, is pull down that End which has the ook in it, to hitch it into the Sling, or he like.

S

SAils Every Yard in the Ship has Sail belonging to it, from which takes its Name The Head-Sails, whic are those belonging to the Fore-Mast an Boltsprit, keep the Ship from the Win and are us'd to flat her The After-Sail that is, the Main-Mast and Mizzen-Sail keep her to the Wind, and therefore fe Ships are so good Condition'd as to ste *Quarter-Winds* with one Sail, but mu have one After-Sail, and another Hea Sail, to countermand one another It common at Sea to call a Ship a Sail, when they spy a Ship, they cry, A Sa A Sail The Sails are cut in Proportio as the Masts and Yards are in Length a Breadth to one another, excepting t Mizzen and Sprit-Sail, for the Mizz Sail is cut by the *Leetch*, twice as deep the Mast is long from the Deck to t Hownds, and the Sprit-Sail is thr Quarters as the Fore-Sail Every o knows, that the Sails are compos'd of veral Breadths of Canvas sew'd togeth according to the Bigness of the Ship, a are, as it were, her Wings, which, wi the Help of the Wind, carry her There have been, and still are, many so of Sails, as well in regard to the Mat they are made of as their Form or Sha The ancient *Gauls* had Sails made of L ther and the Inhabitants of the Island

Borneo use such to this Day The *Chinese* make theirs of Cane, like Masts The People of *Bantam* weave a sort of Grass and Leaves together for this Use The Natives of Cape *Tres Puntas* have Sails made of Straw and Rushes The *Turks* make theirs of Cotton And all the *Europeans* of Sail-Cloth The Sails belonging to a Ship are these; the *Sprit-Sail*, which hangs over the Ship's Head at the Boltsprit, the *Sprit-Sail-Top-Sail*, hanging just over the Sprit-Sail, the *Fore-Sail*, at the Fore-Mast, the *Fore-Top-Sail*, at the Fore-Top-Mast, and the *Fore-Topgallant-Sail*, at the Fore-Topgallant-Mast Then the *Main-Sail*, which is the biggest, at the Main-Mast, the *Main Top-Sail*, over the other at the Main-Top Mast, and the *Main-Topgallant-Sail* over that again at the Main-Topgallant-Mast Lastly, the *Mizzen-Sail*, a-stern at the Mizzen-Mast, and this differs in Shape from all the rest, which are square, and this triangular; and the *Mizzen-Top-Sail* which is like the other Sails Besides these, there are *Stay-Sails*, to crowd in upon Occasion, but these not so common in Use

Sands, are great Banks of Sand in the Sea, dangerous to Ships

To Serve, is to lay Sinnet, Spun-Yarn, Rope-Yarn, a Piece of Canvas, or any such Thing, upon a Rope, and rowl it fast about to keep it from gauling, where there is Danger of their fretting or wearing out against any Part of the Ship

A Scarf, is the End of one Timber let into the End of another, very close and even, or, as the Seamen call it, *Wood and Wood*, that is, as much taken away of the one as of the other So the Stem is fasten'd to the Keel, which is call'd, *the Scarf of the Keel*

Scupper-Holes, Scupper-Leathers, Scupper-Nails Vide *Skuppers*

A Scuttle, is a square Hole, big enough for a Man conveniently to go through, cut through any Hatch, or other Part of the Deck, to go down by into any Room or Part under the Deck Of these, there is one close before the Main Mast, one in the Hatch-way for the Steward's-Room; one in the Gun-Room to go down into the Stern-Sheats, one in the Mizzen-Cabbin to go down into the Captain's Cabbin; and so in other Places Besides, all the little Windows and Holes that are cut out aloft in the Captain's or Master's Cabbins, are call'd Scuttles

The Sea All Men know to be the great Collection of Waters, which separates one Part of the World from another

Sea-Bord, is the Side that is out to Seaward, and fromward the Land

Sea Card Vide *Card*

Sea-Drags, are any Thing that hangs over the Ship in the Sea, as Shirts, Gowns, or the like, and so the Boat, when it is tow'd a-Stern, or any other Thing that hinders the Ship's Way, is called, a Drag.

Sea-Gate, is a Billow or Wave, or the ...ng Surge of the rowling Sea

Seams The Seams of a Ship are the ...ints, or meeting together of the Planks

To Sease, or *Seasing*, is to make fast, or ...nd any Ropes together with some small ...ope-Yarn, Marling, or any Line, as also ... fastening of a Block at the End of a ...endant, Tackle, Fall, Garnet, or the like ... short, the Word Seasing in general sig...fies, binding any Thing together so as ...ey cannot part or slip asunder.

The Boat's Seasing, is a Rope made fast ...o a little Chain or Ring, in Foreship ... the Boat, and by it, in Harbour, they ...ake fast the Boat to the Ship's Side

Sea Yoke When the Sea is so rough, or ...rown, as Seamen call it, that Men can...ot govern the Helm with their Hands, ...en they sease two Blocks to the Helm, ...n each Side one, at the very End of it; ...nd reeving two small Ropes, call'd Falls, ...rough them, which are fasten'd to the ...hip's Sides, and so having Men at each Tackle, they thus govern the Helm by ...em, as they are directed There is al...o another Way, which is, by taking a ...ouble Turn about the End of the Helm ...ith a single Rope, which being belay'd ...st to the Ship's Sides, they therewith ...uide the Helm, and either of these ...ays is call'd a Yoke, or Sea-Yoke to ...teer by

A Seel There is no Difference betwixt ...eeling and Heeling, but that the Heeling is a steady lying down of the Ship on a Side, either a Ground, at an Anchor, or under Sail · And *Se ling*, is a sudden lying down, or tumbling to one Side or the other, when the Sea forsakes her; that is, when the Wave of the Sea is pass'd from under her, faster than she can drive away with it The *Lee-Seel*, is when she rowls to the Leeward, wherein there is no Danger, tho' it be in a great Storm, because the Sea will presently come under and right her; but when she rowls back to Windward, the Danger is lest she should come over, too short and suddenly, and so the Water break right into and founder her So that Seeling is but a sudden Heeling

To Send When a Ship, either under Sail, or at an Anchor, falls with her Head or with her Stern deep in the Trough of the Sea, they say, she Sends much either a-Stern or a-Head The Reason of Sending with her Head is, her having a little Bow not sufficient to bear her up, and a fat Quarter to pitch her forward; and so for her Sending a-Stern, it is contrary, when she has too lank a Quarter, and too full a Bow

Serpentine Powder Vide *Powder*

To Set the Land, the Sun, or the Ships, by the Compass, is to observe by the Compass how the Land bears upon any Point of the Compass, and is commonly us'd when a Ship is going out to Sea from any Land, to mark how the Land bears off from them, for the keeping the better Ac-

Account, and directing their Course. They also use to Set the Sun by the Compass, and that is, to observe upon what Point the Sun is at that Time, and so to know the Hour of the Day Besides, when two Ships sail in Sight of one another, and especially when a Man of War chases another Ship, they will Set her by the Compass, that is mark her upon what Point she bears · Then if they stand both one Way, as commonly they do, and the Chased strives to make away, by this it is known whether the Chaser gets upon her or no, for if the Chaser brings her forward on, she out-sails her, if aft, the Chaser is out-sail'd, and if she alter not, then they both go alike

Set the Mizzen, is, fit the Mizzen-Sail

Set-Bolts Vide *Bolts*

Set taught the Shrowds, is, hale or pull them so as they may hang tighter, or not so loose

To Settle a Deck, is to lay it lower than it was

Sewing, or *to Sew*. When the Water is gone from the Ship, so that she lies dry, they say, the Ship is Sew'd, or if it be but gone from any Port at her Head, they say, the Ship is Sew'd a-Head If it be a Place where the Water ebbs so much, that the Ship may lie dry round, then they say, she cannot Sew there

Shackles, are a sort of Rings, tho' not round, but somewhat longish and larger at one End than the other, in the Middle of

 the

the Ports, on the one Side. They are us'd to ſhut faſt the Ports with a Billet, which ſerves for a Bar to them There are others of the ſame Faſhion, but ſmall ones, made faſt to the Corners of the Hatches, to lift them up by

A Shallop Vide *Boat*

The Shank, is the longeſt Part of the Anchor, being that which runs from the Arms to the Ring and Beam

Shank Painter, is a ſhort Chain, faſten'd under the Fore-Maſt-Shrowds, with a Bolt to the Ship's Side, and at the other End has a Rope Upon the Chain reſts the whole Weight of the after-part of the Anchor, when it lies by the Ship's Side; and the Rope by which it is hal'd up is made faſt about a Timber-Head This is ſeldom or never us'd at Sea, but only in Harbour, or a Road

The Sheats; are bent to the Clew of all the Sails, and in all the low ones ſerve to hale aft the Clew of the Sail, but in Top-ſails to hale home, that is, hale cloſe the Clew of the Sail to the Yard Arms When they hale aft the Sheat of the Fore-Sail, it is to make her fall off from the Wind When the Ship will not fall off from the Wind, they flat in the Fore-Sheat, that is, pull the Sail flat in by the Sheat, as near to the Ship's Side as may be *Eaſe the Sheat*, is, veer out, or let go a little of it *Let fly the Sheat*; is, let it run out as far as it will, and then the Sail will hold no Wind, but hang floating looſe hoſe Thoſe Planks under Water, which come along the Run of the Ship, and are cloſ'd to the Stern-Poſt, are alſo call'd Sheats, and that Part within Board, abaft, in the Run of the Ship, is call'd, the *Stern Sheats*

Sheathing, is caſing a Ship, or covering all that is under Water, or a very little above, with Boards, and Hair and Tar laid betwixt the Ship's Sides and thoſe Boards, the Uſe of it being to keep the Worms from eating through the Planks, as is frequent in the Southern Parts The thinner the Boards, the better, for then the Worm comes preſently to the Tar, which it cannot abide, and therefore cannot faſten upon the Plank There has been Sheathing with thin Lead, but that is more chargeable, and heavy

Sheer-Hooks, are great Iron Hooks, in the Nature of ſmall Sickles, ſet into the Arms of the Main and Fore-Yards, the Uſe of them, to tear and cut the Sails and Shrowds of another Ship that ſhall come to Board under Sail, but they are little uſ'd, being very dangerous for breaking of their own Yards, if the Hook ſhould chance to catch in the other Ship's Maſt or Yard

Sheering; is when a Ship in her ſailing is not ſteddily ſteer'd, but goes in and out And where a Tide-Gate runs very ſwift, the Ship will ſheer in and out, and ſo much in ſome Places, that they are fain to have one ſtand at the Helm to ſteer her upon the Tide, for fear she may sheer her Anchors home, or sheer aground, if she is near the Shore

Sheers, are two Masts, Yards or Poles, set up an End a good Distance from each other at Bottom, and seas'd across one another near the Top To this Seasing is fasten'd a double Block, with a Strap, and they are plac'd below upon the Chain-Wales of the Shrowds, and lash'd fast to the Ship's Sides, to keep them steddy a-loft Their Use is either to set in a Mast, or take it out, or else they serve to hoise Goods in or out of Boats that have no Masts

Sheevers There are two Sorts of them, either of Brass or Wood, the Brass ones little us'd, but in the Heels of the Top-Masts; the Wooden ones are either of one whole Piece, and these they use for all small Pullies and small Blocks, but in the Knights and the Winding-Tackle Blocks, they use Sheevers made of Quarters of Wood, let into one another, because they will hold, when the whole Sheevers will split

A Ship, is well known to be a Vessel made of Timbers and Planks, fit to float upon the Water, and to make Way by the Help of its Masts, Rigging, Yards and Sails

A Ship of Charge; is one that draws much Water, sometimes one that is unweildy at Sea, so call'd, because she is dangerous, or a Ship of great Burden

Sheal-

Shoal-Keel Vide *Keel*

Shoaling When the Water, coming towards the Shore, grows ſhallow by Degrees, and not too ſuddenly, nor is ſometimes deep and ſometimes ſhallow; and it is ſafe and commodious going in with the Shore This is call'd good Shoaling, and ſo the contrary is bad

To Shooe the Anchor, is to put Boards to the Flooks, in the ſame Form of them, to make them broader than they were, which is done where the Ground is ſo ſoft and owzie that the Anchors cannot hold

The Shore, is the Land next the Sea, or the Bank of the Sea, the Lee-Shore, that on which the Wind blows, the Weather-Shore, that from whence the Wind comes

Shores, are any Pieces of Timber or other Thing ſet to bear up another from ſinking or falling Alſo ſome Timbers ſet to bear up a Deck, when it is weak, or over-charg'd with Weight, are call'd Shores

Shot There are ſeveral Sorts of it; the Round flies fartheſt, and pierces moſt; the next is Croſs-Bar, good to deſtroy Ropes, Sails and Maſts, a third Langrel, which will not fly ſo far, but tears Rigging, and makes Havock among Men; ſo is Caſe-Shot and Chain-Shot, being proper to ply it among Men that ſtand expos'd to the ſmall Shot.

A Shot of Cable, is two Cables ſplic'd together; the Uſe of them in very deep Wa-

Waters and great Roads, becauſe a Ship rides eaſier by one ſuch Shot, than by three ſhort Cables Vide *Ride*

Showl, and *Shallow*, is one and the ſame Thing

Showling Vide *Shoaling*

Shrowds, are thoſe Ropes which come from either Side the Tops of the Maſts down to the Ship's Sides, and are like Ladders to go up to the Tops There are the Fore, Main, and Mizzen-Shrowds, having at the lower End Dead-Mens Eyes ſeaz'd to them, and are ſet up taught by Lanniers to the Chains, which have alſo Dead-Mens-Eyes in them At the other End they are faſten'd over the Head of the Maſt, the Pendants, Fore-Tackle and Swifters, being firſt put on under them. At this uppermoſt Part they are ſew'd, to prevent gauling againſt the Maſt The Top-Maſt-Shrowds are in like manner faſten'd with Dead-Mens-Eyes and Lanniers to the Puttocks and the Plates of Iron that belong to them, and then again aloft over the Head of the Top-Maſt. *Eaſe*, or, *Slack the Shrowds*, is to let them a little looſer, when they are too ſtiff ſet up *Set taught the Shrowds*, or, *Set up the Shrowd*, is to draw them tighter, when too looſe.

Sidnet, or *Sinnet*, is a Line or String made of Rope-Yarn, of two, ſix, or nine, platted one over another, and ſo beaten ſmooth and flat with a Mallet The Uſe of it is to ſarve Ropes; that is, to wind

wind about them, to keep them from wearing

The Skeg, is that little Part of the Keel which is cut ſlanting, and left a little without the Stern-Poſt The Deſign and Uſe of it is to keep the Rudder from beating off, if the Ship happen to be aground Yet theſe Skegs are very uſeleſs and inconvenient, for they are apt to ſnap off, and ſo endanger the Stern-Poſt Beſides, in a Harbour or River, where many Ships ride, they are apt to catch another Ship's Cable betwixt them and the Rudder Laſtly, when a Ship is under Sail, they hold much dead Water betwixt them and the Rudder Wherefore it is better to have no Skeg, but to hang the Rudder down cloſe to the Stern-Poſt, with the Bottom even to the Bottom of the Keel, only par'd away a little towards the aftermoſt Side of it

Skiff Vide *Boat*

Skuppers, or *Skupper-Holes*, are the Holes cloſe to all the Decks, through the Ship's Sides, through which the Water runs out of the Ship from the Decks

Skupper-Leathers, are the round Leathers nail'd over the Skupper-Holes, that belong to the lower Deck, which keep out the Sea-Water from coming in, and yet let any Water run out from the Deck They are alſo over the Skuppers of the Manger

Skupper-Nails, are little ſhort Nails, with broad Heads, made on purpoſe to nail

nail on the Skupper-Leathers; and with the ſame they nail on the Coats of the Maſts and Pumps

A Slatch When any Part of a Cable or Rope, that is, of the Middle, not the End, hangs ſlack without the Ship in the Water, or looſe by the Ship's Side, they call that, *a Slatch*, and ſay, *Hale up the Slatch of the Rope or Cable* So when it has been a Fit of foul Weather, and there comes an Interval or ſhort Time of fair Weather to ſerve their Turn, they call it, *a Slatch of fair Weather*, or the contrary

Sleepers, are thoſe Timbers which lie fore and aft the Bottom of the Ship, on either Side the Keelſon, as the Rung-Heads do go The lowermoſt of theſe is bolted to the Rung-Heads, and the uppermoſt to the Futtocks; and ſo between them they ſtrengthen and bind faſt the Futtocks and the Rungs, which are let down one by another, and have no other Binding but the Sleepers

Slings The firſt Sort of them is to ſling Casks in, or the like, which are made of a Rope ſplic'd at either End into it ſelf, making an Eye at either End, large enough to receive into it the Cask, and then they ſeaze together the middle Part of the Rope, and ſo make another Eye to hitch in the Hook of the Tackle or Garnet Another Sort of Slings are made long, with a ſmall Eye at either End, to put the one over the Breech of a Gun, the other to come over the End of an Iron Crow, which is put into the Mouth of the Piece, and so by them they hoise it in A third Sort is any Rope or Chain wherewith they bind fast the Yards aloft to the Cross-Trees, and the Head of the Mast; to the end, that if the Ties should break, the Yards may not come down These *Slings* are us'd in Time of Fight, for fear of cutting the Ties

To Sling, is to make fast any Cask, Gun, Yard, or the like, in a Pair of Slings

Smalcraft This Word signifies all Lines, Nets and Hooks, that serve for catching of Fish; as also all small Vessels, such as Ketches, Hoys, and the like

A Smitting-Line, is a small Rope made fast to the Mizzen-Yard-Arm, below next the Deck, and when the Mizzen-Sail is furthel'd up, this is made up alongst with it to the upper End of the Yard, the Sail being made up with Rope-Yarns, and so comes down to the Poop The Use of it is to loose the Mizzen-Sail, without striking down the Yard, for they pull the Rope, which breaks all the Rope-Yarns, and the Sail comes down

A Snatch-Block, is a great Block with a Sheever in it, and a Notch cut through one of the Cheeks of it, by which Notch they reeve any Rope into it, and this is for Quickness to reeve the Rope in, for by this Notch they may reeve the middle Part of the Rope into the Block, without passing it in by the End, which would be be longer a doing It is generally made fast with a Strap about the Main-Mast, close to the upper Deck, and is chiefly us'd for the Fall of the Winding-Tackle, which is reev'd in the Block, and so brought to the Capstain

Sockets The Holes into which the Pintles of the Murderers, Fore-locks, or the like, are plac'd, are call'd Sockets, and some call the Gudgins, in which the Pintles of the Rudder hang, by the same Name

A Sound, is any great Indraught of the Sea, betwixt two Head-Lands, where there is no Passage through, as *Plimouth* Sound, &c But when we say absolutely the Sound, it is meant of that Sea betwixt *Germany*, *Denmark* and *Sweden*, which is the greatest we know of, otherwise call'd the *Baltick* Sea

To Sound, is to try the Depth of the Water with a Line or Pole, or any Way whatever So when they would know what Water is in the Well of the Pump they put down a small Line with a Weight to it, and that is call'd, Sounding the Pump Vide *Deep-Sea-Lead* When they would Sound, the Expression us'd is, *Heave the Lead*

The Sounding-Lead, is as the Deep-Sea Lead for Sounding, but it is commonly only 7 Pounds Weight, and about 12 Inches long

The Sounding-Line The Difference betwixt this and the Deep-Sea-Line, is this

the

the Sounding-Line is bigger than the Deep-Sea-Line. It is commonly cut to twenty Faddom, or little more; whereas the other is an Hundred, or two Hundred. The one is us'd in showl, the other in deep Water The Deep-Sea-Line is first mark'd at twenty Faddom, and so to thirty, forty, &c but the Sounding-Line is mark'd at two Faddom next the Lead, with a Piece of Black Leather put into it betwixt the Strands, and the like at three Faddom, at five, a Piece of White Woollen Cloth, at seven Faddom, a Piece of Red Cloth; at ten, a Piece of Leather; at fifteen Faddom, either a White Cloth, or a Piece of Leather, and then it is mark'd no farther This may be us'd under Sail, but the Deep-Sea-Line cannot with any Certainty

Spar-Deck . Vide *Deck*

Speeks, are like great Iron Pins, with flat Heads, and of several Lengths, as some a Foot or two long, some of them are ragged, that they may not draw out again They are us'd in many Places for fastening of Timbers and Planks In foul Weather, they use to speek up the Guns; that is, nail down a Quoin to the Deck, close to the Breech of the Carriage, to help keep up the Piece strong to the Ship's Side, lest it should break loose when the Ship rowls

A Spell, is a Turn, or certain Time of working, or plying any Labour, and so giving over for others to succeed in

Course;

Courſe: So when they pump an Hundred Strokes, or a Glaſs, they call it, a Spell. *A Freſh Spell*, is others to come to take their Turn for ſuch a Time at the Work. This Word is commonly us'd only for Pumping and Rowing.

To Spell. When a Sail has much Wind in it, and they would let the Wind out of it, either to take it in, or for fear of wronging the Maſts, they ſay, *Spell the Sail*, and this is done by letting go the Sheats and Bowlings, and bracing the Weather-Brace in the Wind. Then the Sail will lie all looſe in the Wind. This Word is moſt commonly us'd to the Mizzen-Sail, for when they take it in, or ſpeek it up, they ſay, *Spell the Mizzen*.

To Spend; is to break; for they ſay they have ſpent their Maſt or Yard, when it is broke by foul Weather, or the like. But if this happen in Fight, they do not uſe the Word Spent, but ſhot by the Board, or carry'd away by the Board with a Shot, or with another Ship's Maſts or Yards, that is bigger or ſtronger.

Spiked; is when Iron Nails or Spikes are drove into the Touch-hole of a Gun by an Enemy, which makes it unfit for Service.

The Spindle, is the ſmalleſt Part of the Capſtain, which is betwixt the two Decks. To the Spindle of the Jeer-Capſtain, there are Whelps to heave the Viol.

To Splice, is to make faſt the Ends of Ropes one into another, by opening the Strand

Strands at the Ends of both Ropes, and then, with a Fid, laying every Strand orderly one into another Also when an Eye is to be made at the End of any Rope, they undo the Strands at the End of the Rope with a Fid, and draw them into the Ends of the other, and so weaving them orderly, make a Splice, and sease the Ends down with some Sinnet, or the like There are these Sorts of Splices The round Splice, that is, the splicing the Ends of two Ropes one into another, as has been describ'd, and the Cunt-Splice, which is, when the End of one Rope is splic'd into another Rope, at some Distance from the End, and not one End into another, like the first Then they will make a long Slit, as it were betwixt them, wh[illegible] is the Reason of the Name.

Split When the Wind has blown a Sail in Pieces, they say, *The Sail is split*; and so when the Sheevers break, they say, they split. And if a Shot breaks the Carriage of a Gun, they say, it has split the Carriage

To Spoon, or *Spooning*; is putting a Ship right before the Wind and the Sea, without any Sail, which is call'd, Spooning afore, which is commonly done when in a great Storm a Ship is so weak, with Age or labouring, that they dare not lay her under the Sea Sometimes, to make a Ship go the steadier, they set the Fore-Sail, which is call'd, *Spooning with the Fore-Sail* They must be sure of Sea-Room enough when they do this

To Spring When a Mast is only crack'd in any Part, as at the Hownds, Partners, or elsewhere, they say, *it is sprung* *To spring a Leak*, is when with Stress of Weather something gives Way, and lets in the Water *To spring ones Loof* Vide *Loof*

The Spring, or *Spring-Tide*, is when, after the Dead-Neaps, the Tides begin to rise and run higher, and this begins about three Days before the Full and Change of the Moon, and the Top or Highest of the Spring is three Days after Then the Water swells highest with the Flood, and falls lowest with the Ebb, and they run much stronger and swifter than in the Neaps And this is the Time to launch and grave Ships

To spring a-But, is when a Plank is loose at one End, for a *But* is properly the End of a Plank joining to another, on the outside of a Ship under Water

Sprit Sail Vide *Sail*

Sprit-Sail-Top-Sail Vide *Sail*

Sprit-Sail-Top-Mast Vide *Mast*.

Sprit-Sail-Yard Vide *Yard*

A Spunge, is that which makes a Gun clean within, both before charging and after firing In Fight, to keep the Gun from heating, they wet the Spunges with Urine, Vinegar, Water, or such as they have The Spunge is made of Sheep-skins, lapp'd about the End of a Staff, so thick, that it may go in full and close but not too streight.

Spun

Spun-Yarn, is Rope-Yarn, the End scrap'd thin, and so spun one to the End of another with a Wrench, so to make it as long as they please, and is us'd to saive Ropes with, and also to make Caburn of

Sparkets, are the Holes or Spaces betwixt the *Futtocks* or the *Rungs* by the Ship's Sides, fore and aft, below and above There are Boards fitted to the *Spurkets* which are below the Sleepers, in the Hould, which they take up to clear the Spurkets if any Ballast get between the Timbers But for those aloft, there is no Use

Standing-Parts of Running Ropes, are those Parts of Running Ropes, or rather the Ends of them, which are any where made fast to the Ship, to distinguish them from the other Parts by which they use to hale So when they say, *Hale the Sheat*, that is meant by the running Part But if they say, *Over-hale the Sheat*, then they hale upon the Standing Part, and the same is to be understood in all Tackles and Running Ropes

Standing-Quoyns Vide *Quoyns*

Standing-Ropes, are all such Ropes as use not to be remov'd, or to run in any Blocks; but only are set taughter or slacker, as they have Occasion, as the *Shrowd-Stays*, and the *Back-Stays*, &c

To Stay, or *bring a Ship to Stay* When the Ship is to tack, before she can be ready so to do, she must come *a-Stays*, or *a-Back-Stays*, at which Time the Wind comes

comes in at the Bow, which before wa
the Lee-Bow, and ſo drives all the Sail
backwards againſt the Maſts and Shrowds
ſo that the Ship has no Way, but drive
with her Broad-Side The Method o
doing it, is all at once to bear up th
Helm, let fly the Sheat of the Fore-Sail, le
go the Fore-Bowling, and brace the Wea
ther-Brace of the Fore-Sail, the Top an
Topgallant-Sail, and keep faſt their Sheat
If the Sprit-Sail be out, they let go th
Sprit-Sail-Sheat with the Fore-Sheat, an
brace the Weather-Brace The Tack
Sheats, Braces, and Bowlings of the Main
Sail, Main-Top-Sail, and Mizzen, ſtan
faſt as they did, to be taken a-Stays

Stays, and *Back-Stays*. All the Maſt
Top-Maſts, and Flag-Staves, have Stay
excepting the Sprit Sail-Top-Maſt Th
Main-Stay is made faſt by a Lannier to
Collar, which comes about the Knee o
the Head The Main-Top-Maſt-Stay
made faſt into the Head of the Fore-Ma
by a Strop and a Dead-Man's-Eye ther
The Main-Topgallant-Maſt is in li
manner made faſt to the Head of t
Fore-Top-Maſt, the Fore-Maſt, and oth
Maſts belonging to it, are in the ſam
manner ſtay'd at the Boltſprit and Spr
Sail-Top-Maſt, and theſe ſame Stays
alſo help to ſave the Boltſprit T
Mizzen-Stay comes to the Main-Maſt
the Half-Deck; and its Top-Maſt-Sta
come to the Shrowds with Crows-Fe
The Uſe of the Stays is to keep the Ma
fro

from falling aftward towards the *Poop* The Back-Stays of all Masts, which have them, being only the Main, and Fore-Mast, and other Masts belonging to them, go down to either Side of the Ship, and are to keep the Masts from pitching forward on over Board

Steady, is a Word us'd by him that conds to the Steersman, which is to keep the Ship from going in and out, or in the Sea *Phrase*, from making Yaws

To Steer, is to govern the Ship with the Helm There are three Sorts of Directions to steer by, the one by the Land, that is, by any Mark on the Land, and so to keep the Ship even by that, and this is easy The next by the Compass, that is, to keep her upon a Point of the Compass, which is harder, because the Ship's Head will come before the Compass The third is to steer to, as they are directed, or conded, which is the easiest of all For the Terms of *Steering*, Vide *Cond.* He steers best, who keeps the Ship evenest from yawing in and out, and uses least Motion in putting the Helm too far over.

The Steeridge, is the Place where they steer, whence they may see the Leetch of the Sails, to perceive whether they be in the Wind or not

The Stem; is that great Timber which comes compassing from the Keel, into which it is scarf'd up before the Fore-castle; and this guides the Rake of the Ship

Ship To give a Ship the Stem is to run right upon her with the Stem To go ſtemming aboard a Ship, is the ſame as giving a Ship the Stem

A Step, is that Piece of Timber which is made faſt to the Keelſon, in which the Main-Maſt ſtands And ſo thoſe are alſo *Steps* in which the Fore-Maſt, the Mizzen-Maſt, and the Capſtain, ſtand

The Stern, is all the aftermoſt Part of the Ship in general, but more particularly, only the outwardmoſt Part abaft is the Stern, the Quarter being counted from the Steeridge to the Tranſome and Faſhion-Piece of the Stern

Stern the Buoy Vide *Buoy*

Stern-Chaſe, is when a Ship is ſo built as to carry many Guns to ſhoot right aft and when ſhe can do this, they ſay, ſhe has a good Stern-Chaſe

A Stern Faſt, is a Cable or Hawſer brought through the Cat-Holes, which are above the Gun-Room Ports a-Stern by which the Ship is heav d a-Stern upon Occaſion

To Steve, or *Steving* When the Boltſprit or Beak-head ſtands too upright, and not ſtrait forward enough, they ſay, it *ſteves* Merchants call ſtowing of their Cottons, which they force in with Skrews ſo hard, that the Decks will riſe ſome Inches, *Steving of Cottons*

The Steward, is an Officer, whoſe Buſineſs it is to receive the whole Maſs of Victuals from the Purſer, to ſee it well

an

and conveniently ſtow'd in the Hould; to look well to it when there, to take into his Cuſtody all the Candles and other Things of that Nature belonging to the Ship; to take Care of the Bread in the Bread-Room; and to ſhare out the Proportions of all the ſeveral Meſſes in the Ship

The Steward's Room, is a peculiar Part in the Hould aſſign'd for the Steward to ſtow the Proviſions, and there he ſleeps and eats

A Stirrop When a Ship by any Miſchance has loſt a Piece of her Keel, and they cannot well come to mend it, but only patch a new Piece into it, they bind it with an Iron, which comes under the Keel, and ſo upon either Side of the Ship, where it is nail'd very ſtrong with Speeks to ſtrengthen it, and this Piece ſo put to the Keel they call a Stirrop

Stoak'd When the Water cannot come to the Well, they ſay, *The Ship is ſtoak'd*; which is, when the *Limber-Holes* are ſtopped with Ballaſt, or any other Thing, ſo that the Water cannot paſs, and then they ſay, *The Limbers are ſtoak'd* Or when any thing is got to the Bottom of the Pump, ſo that it cannot draw Water, they ſay, *The Pump is ſtoak'd*

Stop When they come to an Anchor, and have let run out as much Cable as they think ſufficient to make the Ship ride, or if they be in a Current, where it is beſt to ſtop her a little by Degrees, they ſay, *Stop the Ship*; that is, hold faſt the Cable, and then veer out a little more, and then ſtop her quite to let her ride. For ſtopping Leaks, Vide *Leaks*

A Stopper, is a Piece of Rope with a Wale-Knot at one End, and a Lannier ſplic'd to it, and the other End made faſt to ſome Part, as the Stoppers for the Cables to the Bottom of the Bits by the Deck, the Stoppers of the Main-Halliards to the Knight The Uſe of them is chiefly for the Cables, to ſtop them when they come to an Anchor, that it may go out by little and little, which is done by binding the Wale-Knot about the Cable with the Lanniers, and it will catch hold, ſo that it cannot ſlip away, as the Nippers do, which hold off the Cable The Term us'd in this Caſe is, *laying on the Stoppers*, and *caſting off the Stoppers* They are alſo us'd to the Halliards, when the Yard is hois'd aloft, to ſtop it till the Halliards are belay'd A Ship rides by the Stoppers, when the Cable is not bitted, but only held faſt by them, which is not ſafe riding in a Streſs.

A Storm, is a boiſterous Wind, yet reckoned a Degree lower than a Tempeſt.

To Stow; is to put Goods in Hould in order; for if they be not ſo, they ſay, it is not ſtow'd, but lies in Hould So if any Goods be plac'd in order between the Decks, it is call'd *Stowing* Alſo the placing and laying the Top-Sails in the Top, is call'd *Stowing the Sails*.

A Strake; is a Seam between two Planks, as the *Garboard Strake*; which see in its Place *The Ship heels a Strake*, is when there is the whole Breadth of a Plank rising from the Keel, before they come to the Floor-Timbers

A Strap; is a Rope splic'd about any Block, to make the Block fast by to any Place, where they have Occasion to use it, by the Eye made in the Strap, at the Arse of the Block

A Stream-Anchor, is a small Anchor, us'd to the Stream-Cable Vide *Anchor*.

A Stream-Cable, is a small Cable, to ride by in Streams, in Rivers, or in fair Weather In stopping a Tide, they always use the smallest Ground-Tickle they have, if it will hold, which is done both for Lightness to weigh, and to save the best from wetting

A Stretch When they go to hoise a Yard, or hale the Sheat, they say, *Stretch* forwards the Halliards, or the Sheats, that is, deliver along that Part which they must hale by into the Mens Hands, that they may be ready to hoise or hale.

Stretchers, are only us'd in Boats, and are those Wooden Staves the Rowers set their Feet against when they row, that so they may be able to fetch the stronger Stroke

To Strike, is to let fall the Sails When Ships strike to one another, it is paying Respect, unless it be done to stay for one another. If an Enemy's Ship strikes, it signifies that she yields When a Ship beats upon the Ground, they also say *she strikes* When they take down the Top Masts they call it, *Striking of them* When they lower any Thing into the Hould with the Tackles, or any other Rope, they call it, *Striking down into Hould* The letting the Colours run down upon the Staff, is also call'd, *Striking*.

To Suck When all the Water is drawn out, and the Pump draws Wind, they say, she sucks The same Word is us'd when a Ship draws down the Helm, and and as it were sucks the Whip-Staff out of the Steersman's Hands

A Surge, is a Wave But when they heave at the Capstain, and the Cable slips back again, they say, *The Cable surges*

The Swabber, is the lowest Office aboard a Ship, his Business being to see the Ship kept neat and clean in all Parts, to which End he is, at least once or twice a Week, if not every Day, to cause the Ship to be well wash'd within Board, and without above Water, especially about the Gun-Wales and Chains; and for preventing of Infection to burn sometimes Pitch or any such wholesome Perfumes, between the Decks He is also to have an Eye to every private Man's Sleeping-Place, to warn them all to be cleanly and neat, and to complain to the Captain of all that are nasty

The Sweep, is the Mould in which the Futtocks are plac'd

Swe pi

Sweeping, is hanging a Three-flook'd Grapnel over the Boat's Stern, and letting it down into the Sea or Channel; and by the rowing of the Boat to drag it on the Ground up and down, to find some Cable or Hawser slipp'd from an Anchor, to which no Buoy was fasten'd.

To Swift the Boat, is to make fast a Rope by the Gun Wale round about the Boat, and fasten the Boat-Rope to that, and with this Boat-Rope, the Boat is tow'd at the Ship's Stern, by which Swifting, the Boat is strengthen'd to endure the Tow.

Swifters, belong to the Main and Fore-Mast, and serve to relieve and strengthen the Shrowds, and keep the Mast stiff. They have their Pendants made fast under the Shrowds, at the Head of the Masts, with a double Block, through which is reev'd the Swifter, which at the standing Part has a single Block, with a Hook hitch'd in a Ring by the Chun-Wale, and so being hal'd, does help to strengthen the Masts.

Swifting, is us'd in the Sea Language when Ships are brought on Ground, or to Careen, then they swift the Masts, to ease and strengthen them, which is done by laying fast all the Pendants of the Swifters and Tackles with a Rope, close to the Masts, as near the Blocks as may be, then they carry forward the Tackles, and so bowse them down, that is, hale them down, as hard and taught as possible. This eases the Mast, so that all its Weight does not hang by the Head, as otherwise it would, and it also helps to keep them from rising out of the Steps

T

TAcks, are great Ropes, with a Wale-Knot at one End, which is seas'd into the Clew of the Sail, and so reev'd first through the Chess-Tree, and then comes in at a Hole of the Ship's Side The Use of them is to carry forwards the Clews of the Sails, and make them stand close by a Wind, and then the Sails are thus trimm'd The Main, Fore, and Mizzen Tacks, are close a-Board, or hal'd as forward in as may be, and so are the Bowlings of the Weather-Side · The Lee-Sheats are hal'd close aft, but the Lee-Sheats of the Fore-Sail not so much, unless the Ship gripe The Lee-Braces of all the Yards are brac'd aft, and the Top Sails are govern'd as the Sails they belong to Hence they say, *A Ship sails close under a Tack*, that is, close by a Wind *Hale aboard the Tack*, is to hale it down close to the Chess-Trees *Ease the Tack*, is not quite so close aboard *Let rise the Tack*, is, let it go all out It is commonly belay'd to the Bits, or else there is a Kevel that belongs to them These Tacks only belong to the Main Sail, Fore-Sail, and Mizzen, and are ever made tapering

To Tack a Ship, is to bring her Head about, to lie the other Way, as if her Head at first lay West North-West, now it will lie East-North-East, the Wind being at North. Then supposing a Ship has all her Sails out, which they use by a Wind, they do thus. First, make her Stay, for which, Vide *Stays*, then they say, *She is Pay'd*, and so let the Lee-Tack rise, and hale aft the Sheats, and so trim all her Sails by a Wind, as they were before.

Tackles, are small Ropes, that run in three Parts, having either a Pendant with a Hook to it, or a Rammer, and at the other End a Block and Hook, to catch hold and heave in Goods into the Ship. There are these several Sorts, the Boat's Tackles, which stand one on the Main-Mast-Shrowds, the other on the Fore-Mast-Shrowds, to hoise in the Boat, and they also serve for other Uses. The Tackles which belong to the Mast, which serve in the Nature of Shrowds, to keep the Mast from straining. The Gunner's Tackles, with which they hale the Guns in and out. And, lastly, the Winding-Tackle; which see in its Place. That Part of the Tackle which they hale upon, is call'd, *the Fall*, but the End to which the Block is seaz'd, is call'd, *the Standing Part*. To hale upon the Tackle, is term'd, to bowse upon the Tackle.

To Tally. When they hale aft the Sheats of Main or Fore-Sail, they say, *Tally aft the Sheats*.

Tapering; is when any Rope or other Thing is made bigger at one End than at the other, as the Tacks are made tapering, for which Reason they purchase the better, and it saves a great deal of Stuff, because the Rope at one End bears little or no Stress

Taper Bore; is when the Bore of a Gun is wider at the Mouth than towards the Breech, which Pieces are not good, for if the Shot that goes in at the Mouth will not go home to the Powder, but stick by the Way, it endangers the Gun

Tar-Pawling, is a Piece of Canvas tarr'd all over, to lash upon a Deck or Grating to keep the Rain or other Water from soaking through

Taunt. When a Mast is very high for the Proportion of the Ship, they say, *It is a Taunt Mast*

Taught, is tight, stiff, or fast; as they say, *Set taught the Shrowds, the Stays*, or any other Rope, when it is too slack

A Tempest When it over-blows so exceedingly, that there is no bearing any Sail, and the Wind is mix'd with Rain or Hail, they call it a Tempest, and that is reckon'd a Degree above a Storm

The Thaughts, are the Seats on which they sit who row in the Boat

Thowles, are the small Pins which they bear against with their Oars when they row, and stand in Holes on the upper Side of the Gun-Wale of the Boat; being commonly madeof Ash, for Toughness

Thwart-

Thwart-Ships That is, a-cross the Ship from one Side to the other, the contrary being *alongst Ships*, that is, along the Ship from Head to Stern.

Tide This Word is pretty well known to all Men, and is common to the Ebb and Flood, which are call'd, *Tide of Ebb*, and *Tide of Flood* *A Windward Tide*, is when the Tide runs against the Wind, at which Time the Sea breaks most, and runs highest, but then a Ship at Anchor strains the Cables least *A Leeward Tide*, is when the Wind and Tide go both one Way, then the Sea is smoother When they say, *It flows Tide and Half-Tide in any Place*, which is a very improper Expression, the Meaning is, that the Tide runs three Hours, which is four Points longer in the Offing than it does by the Shore, that is, if it be High-Water at the Shore at twelve a Clock, it will not be High-Water in the Offing till three, which is the Time for the Running of half a Tide; So as it ebbs or flows more, they say, *It runs Tide* When they come into Harbour they say, they will bring their Tide with them; that is, come in with the Flood, to carry them over any Showls

A Tide-Gate, is where the Tide runs very strong

To Tide over, or up to a Place, is to go with the Tide of Flood or Ebb, and to stop the contrary Tide at an Anchor, till the same Tide come again, which is us'd when the Wind is contrary, but does not over-blow

The Ties; are Four-ſtrand Ropes, Hawſer-laid, becauſe this ſort of Laying does not ſtretch ſo much as the Three-ſtrand Ropes, and runs ſmoother in the Hownds By theſe Ropes the Yards hang, and they carry up the Yards, when the Halliards are ſtrain'd to hoiſe the Yards The Main and Fore-Yard Ties are firſt reev'd through the Ram-Head, then through the Hownds at the Head of the Maſt, and ſo with a Turn in the Eyes of the Slings, which are made faſt to the Yard, they are ſeaz'd faſt and cloſe to the Yard The Mizzen-Yard and Top-Maſt-Yard have but ſingle Ties The Sprit-Sail has one made faſt with a Pair of Slings to the Boltſprit

The Tiller, is the ſame as the Helm Vide *Helm* Only the Word Tiller is moſt properly us'd for that they ſteer the Boat by, and ſo they ſay, *Hand me the Tiller of the Boat*, and not the Helm, tho' the Uſe of both be the ſame

Tight When a Ship is Staunch and makes but little Water, ſhe is then Tight, and this is ſoon known by the Smell of the Water, for if it ſtink much, it is a Sign it has lain long in the Ship, and if it is ſweet, that it is newly come in

The Tilt, is a Covering to ſpread over a Boat, ſupported on Hoops or Bales, to keep off the Sun in [illegible] Weather, or the Rain from thoſe wh[illegible] it

A Tire, is, as we may ſay, a whole Round, or Guns every where fore and aft on the Deck Some Ships have two

or

or three Tires of Guns The Fore-Castle and the Half-Deck being furnish'd, make half a Tire *The Cable Tire*, is the Space that is in the Middle of the Cable, when it it is quoil'd up

Tompions, are Bits of Wood, turn'd fit for the Mouths of the Guns, and put into them, to keep out the Rain or Sea-Water from washing in, when the Mouths lie without Board

Top-Armours, are the Cloths that are ty'd about the Tops of the Masts for Show, as also to hide Men that lie there in Time of Fight, to fling Fire-Pots, ply small Shot, or the like

Topgallant-Masts, are the Masts above the Top-Masts Vide *Masts* And only the Main and Fore-Masts have them

Topgallant-Sails, are the Sails at the Topgallant-Masts Vide *Sails* And these Sails draw Quarter-Winds very much in a Loom or fresh Gale, so it blows not too much

Top-Masts, are generally half as long as the Masts they belong to, and stand on their Heads They belong to the Fore, Main, and Mizzen Masts

Top-Ropes, are those wherewith they set or strike the Top Masts, and belong only to the Main and Fore-Top-Masts They are reev'd through a great Block, that is seiz'd under the Cap on one Side, and then it is reev'd through the Heel of the Top-Mast, where there is a Brass Sheever plac'd a-thwart Ships, and then brought up and made fast on either Side of the Cap, with a Clinch to a Ring, which is fasten'd into the Cap The other Part comes down by the Ties, and is reev'd into the Knight and brought to the Capstain, when they heave it

Tops, are the Round, as it were, Floors made at the Top of all Masts, for Men to stand on, being made of Boards, and strengthen'd round with Iron

Top-Sails; are those that belong to the Top-Masts Vide *Sails*

Top the Lifts, or *Top the Martnets*; is no other than hale them.

To Tow, is to drag any thing at the Ship's Stern in the Water. The nearer any Thing is when tow'd, the less it hinders the Ship's Way, but the farther off, the easier it is for that which is tow'd, because then the Ship does not give such Twitches

The Transome, is the Timber that lies a-thwart the Stern of the Ship, betwixt the two Fashion-Pieces, and lays out her Breadth at the Buttock 'Tis just under the Gun-Room-Port a-Stern *To lie with a Ship's Transome*, is to lie just with the End of the Planks, where they are fasten'd to the Fashion-Pieces a-Stern *To come in with a Ship's Transome*, is just betwixt her Gun-Room-Port and her Quarter-Port, and this is the safest coming up, because there Ships are most naked, and there Gallies use to come up with Ships

Traverse. The Way of the Ship, in respect of the Points whereon they sail, and the Angles the Ship makes in going to and again, is the Traverse of the Ship.

To Traverse a Yard; is to set it any way over-thwart

To Traverse a Gun; is to lay and remove it, till it comes to bear with the Mark

Traverse-Boord; is a Boord kept in Steeridge, on which the 32 Points of the Compass are mark'd, with little Holes at every Point, for him at the Helm to keep a Score, how many Glasses they have gone upon a Point of the Compass, and so strike in a Pin at that Point, which is to save the Master a Labour, who cannot so nicely watch every Wind and Course as he at the Helm, especially when they go by a Wind, and the Wind veers and heels

To Trench the Ballast Vide *Ballast*

The Trenels, signify as much as Nails made of Tree, being long Wooden Pins made of the Heart of Oak, wherewith they fasten all the Planks to the Timbers; for tho' they bolt the Bulk-Head, for the better Assurance and Strength, yet the Trenels are the Things that most fasten the Planks; because they use as little Iron under Water as possible, lest the Ship grow Iron-sick These Trenels must be well season'd, and not sappy, for then the Ship will be continually leaky, and it will be hard to find the Occasion If a Ship by any beating upon the Ground makes a give-back, and comes a little

out

out again, they term it, *Starting of a Tre-nel*

The Treffel-Trees, are join'd to the Cross-Trees, and they lie a-cross each other, and serve to the same Use ; the only Difference being, that the Treffel-Trees are those which go alongst Ships, and the others athward Ships. Vide *Cross-Trees*

Trice, is to hale up any Thing with a Dead-Rope, that is, a Rope which does not run in any Block, but only by Hand

To Try, or *Trying*, is to have no Sail out but the Main-Sail, the Tacks aboord, the Bowling set up, the Sheat close aft, and the Helm ty'd down close aboard Some try with only their Mizzen, but that is only when it blows so much, that they cannot maintain the Main-Sail

The Trim. By this Word is commonly understood the swimming of her, either a Head or a-Stern, or on an even Keel, and in which of these the Ship goes best, that they call her Trim Yet this is not only to be counted her Trim, for some Ships will go well or ill according to the Staying of the Masts, the Slackness of the Shrowds, or the like Therefore, in some Men's Opinions, the Order of this Swimming consider'd with this fitting of her Masts and Ropes, wherein the Ship sails best, should be reckon'd her Trim, and not only the Line of her swimming in Water The Ways of finding Ships Trim, must be by sailing with another Ship, to bring her a-Head so many Glasses, then

then a-Stern as many, and then on an even Keel That Way which ſhe goes beſt, is her Trim

A-Trip When the Top-Sails are hois'd to the higheſt, they ſay, they are *a-Trip*

The Trough of the Sea, is the Hollow betwixt two Waves. When they lay a Ship under the Sea, that is, her Broad-Side to the Sea, they ſay, *She lies in the Trough of the Sea*

Trucks; are the little Wooden Wheels without any Spokes, that the Carriages of the Guns run on Alſo thoſe round Things of Wood, which belong to the Parcels, are call'd Trucks

Trunnions, are the Knobs which come from the Sides of the great Guns, and bear them up on the Cheeks of the Carriages

Truſſes, are Ropes made faſt to the Parcel of the Yards, and ſerve for two Uſes; one to bind faſt the Yard to the Maſt when ſhe rowls, either a-Hull, or at an Anchor; the other to hale down the Yards in a Storm Theſe belong only to the Main, Mizzen, and Fore-Yard

The Tuck, is the gathering up of the Ship's Quarter under Water If it lie low, that makes the Ship have a fat Quarter, and hinders the Water from paſſing ſwiftly to the Rudder If it lie high, the Ship muſt be well laid out in the Quarter, elſe ſhe will want Bearing for her after Works, which being ſo high and heavy, charge a Ship very much

A Turn Vide *Boord*

V

TO *Veer out a Rope*, is to put it out by Hand, or let it run out when they may ſtop it, as, *Veer out more Cable*, that is, let more run out It is generally us'd for veering out of thoſe Ropes which are us'd without Board, as to the Boat-Rope, the Log-Line, or the like; but it is not us'd to any running Rope, except only the Sheats When the Wind goes in and out, that is, ſometimes to one Point, and ſometimes to another, and that on a ſudden, as it is apt to do in Storms, they ſay, *the Wind does veer and hull*

Veering When a Ship ſails, and the Sheat is veer'd out, they ſay, *ſhe goes veering* Vide *Large*, and *Quarter-Winds*, which all come to the ſame.

Under-Metal, ſignifies, that the Mouth of a Gun lies lower than the Breech.

A Viol. When the Main-Capſtain is not able to purchaſe in the Cable, by reaſon that the Anchor is let fall into ſuch ſtiff Ground, that they cannot weigh it, or elſe the Sea runs ſo high, that it cannot purchaſe it in, then for more Help they take a Hawſer, and open one Strand of it, and ſo put in it Nippers, ſome ſix or eight, about a Faddom Diſtance from each other, and with theſe Nippers, which are ſmall Ropes with a little Truck at one End, they bind faſt the

the Hawser to the Cable, and then bring it to the Jeer-Capstain, and heave upon it; and this will purchase more than the Main-Capstain can And this Viol is fasten'd together at both Ends with an Eye and a Wale-Knot, or else with two Eyes seaz'd together

W.

A *Wad*, is any Thing ramm'd down into a Gun to keep the Shot close to the Powder, and prevent its rowling out.

To Waft, is what we generally call to convoy, that is, to conduct and guard any Ship or Fleet at Sea: Hence

Wafters; is a Word us'd for Men of War

A-Waift, is a Sign for the Boat to come aboard, and is a Coat, Gown, or the like, hung up in the Shrowds When a Ship hangs a-Waift upon the Main-Stay, it is a Sign of Distress, as that it has sprung a-Leak, or the like

The Wake, is the smooth Water which the Ship makes a-Stern of her, showing the Way she has gone in the Sea. By this they give a Judgment what Way the Ship does make; for if the Wake be right a-Stern, then they reckon she makes her Way good as she looks, but if the Wake be a Point, two or more, to Leeward, then the Ship goes to Leeward of her Course When the Ship does stay a-Weather of her Wake, that is, when in her

her ſtaying ſhe does it ſo quickly, that ſhe does not fall to the Leeward, and when ſhe is tack'd her Wake is to the Leeward, it is a ſure Sign that the Ship feels her Helm well, and is nimble of Steerage In chaſing, when the Chaſer is gotten as far into the Wind as the Chas'd, and ſo ſails directly after her, then they ſay, *they have gotten her Wake*

Wale Vide *Bend*

A Wale-Knot, is a round Knot or Knob, made with three Strands of a Rope, ſo that it cannot ſlip, and with theſe Wale-Knots, the Tacks, the Top-Sail-Sheats, and the Stoppers, are made faſt; as are ſome other Ropes beſides.

Wale-Rear'd; is when a Ship is built right up, after ſhe comes to her Bearing, which is unſightly, and, as the Seamen term it, not Ship-ſhapen; but it makes a Ship within Board much the roomer, and not the leſs wholeſome in the Sea, if her Bearing be well laid out

Walt A Ship is ſaid to be Walt, when ſhe has not Ballaſt enough to keep her ſtiff to bear a Sail

The Wap; is that wherewith the Shrowds are ſet taught There are alſo ſmall Waps, which are ſeaz'd to the midſt of the Top-Maſt, and Topgallant-Stay

A Warp; is any Rope us'd to warp a Ship, and is moſt commonly a Hawſer

To Warp; is to have a Hawſer, or any other Rope ſufficient to hale up a Ship and

and an Anchor bent to it, and ſo lay that out over the Bar over which they are to go, and by that hale the Ship forwards. It is us'd when they want a Wind to carry them out, or into a Harbour; and this is call'd *Warping*.

To Waſh a Ship, is us'd at Sea, when they cannot come a-ground, or careen her They make her heel over to a Side with her Guns, and Men on the Yard-Arms, and ſo waſh that Side and ſcrape it, as far as out of the Water, which is commonly five or ſix Strakes; and this is done in Calms, or in a ſmooth Road.

To Waſh off the Shore; that is, cloſe by the Shore

Waſte, is that Part of the Ship which is between the Main-Maſt and the Fore-caſtle

Waſte-Boards; are the Boards that are ſet up in the Waſte of a Ship, betwixt the Gun-Wale and the Waſte-Trees, but moſt us'd in Boats, to be ſet up alongſt the Sides, to keep the Sea from breaking into them

Waſte-Cloths, are all thoſe which are round about the Cake-Work of the Hull of the Ship, being the ſame they call by another Name, the Fights of the Ship.

Waſte-Trees; are thoſe Pieces of Timber which lie in the Waſte of a Ship

Watch At Sea, the Ship's Company is divided into two Parts, the one call'd the Starboard, and the other the Larboard Watch The Maſter is the Chief of the

Star-

Starboard, and his first Mate of the Larboard These are in their Turns to watch, trim Sails, pump and do all Duties for four Hours, and then the other Watch relieves them for the same Time, which they do throughout the whole Day and Night Four Hours they call a whole Watch In Roads and Harbours, they watch by Quarter-Watch, that is, when only one Quarter of the Ship's Company watches at a Time

Water-Borne. When a Ship is just off the Ground, so that she floats, she is said to be *Water-Borne*

The Water-Line, is the Line which Shipwrights pretend should be the Depth for the Ship to swim in, when she is laden both a-Head and a-Stern; for a Ship never draws so much a-Head as she does a-Stern, because if she did, she could never steer well

Water-Shot; is a Way of Mooring, laying the Anchors, neither a-cross the Tide, nor right up and down with it, but betwixt both, or Quartering

The Water-Way, is the small Ledge or Piece of Timber which lies fore and aft on the Ship's Deck, close by the Sides, to keep the Water from running down there

Waving; is making a Sign for a Ship or Boat to come towards, or go from them, as the Sign is made, either towards or fromwards the Ship.

Way of a Ship The Rake and Run of the Ship are call'd her Way forward on, or aftward on When a Ship sails apace, they say, *she has good Way*, *fresh Way*, or the like In casting a Dead-Reckoning, they allow a Leeward-Way, which is as much as she drives to Leeward from the Way she seems to go

To Weather; is to go to Windward of a Place or Ship.

Weather-Bow, is the Bow next the Weather, and so of all other Parts of the Ship, as the Weather-Side, or any Thing that is to the Windwardmost-Side, they call it the Weather-Part, or a-Weather

Weather-Coile; is when a Ship is a-Hull, to lay her Head the other Way, without loosing any Sail, which is done by only bearing up the Helm, and that is an excellent condition'd Ship which will do it, for most Ships will not *Weather-Coile* The Use of it is, that when they would drive with her Head the other Way, a-Hull, they need not open any Sail, wherewith before the Ship can come to veer, she will run a great Way to Leeward, when once she is before the Sea under Sail.

Wedges; are us'd to make fast the Mast in the Partners. They also put a Wedge into the Heels of the Top Masts, to bear them upon the Tressel-Trees

Wending; is the turning about of a Ship when she is at Anchor.

The Whelps; are like Brackets, set to the Body of the Capstain, close under the Bars, down to the Deck, and serve to give the Sweep to the Capstain They are made so in Parts, that the Cable may not be so apt to surge as it would, if it were to run upon a Body entirely round

A Wherry; is one of the smallest Sort of Boats

The Whip; is the Staff the Steersman holds in his Hand wherewith he governs the Helm, and ports it over from one Side to the other. It has a Ring at one End, which is put over the End of the Helm, and so comes through the Rowl up into the Steeridge. Whips are not us'd in great Ships, because, by Reason of the great Weight of the Rudder, and the Water which lies upon it in foul Weather, they are not able to govern the Helm with a Whip, but one Man being able to stand to it conveniently.

Wholesom.. A Ship is said to be wholesome at Sea, when she will Hull, Try and Ride well, without rowling or labouring much in the Sea

Whoodings, are the Planks which are join'd and fasten'd alongst the Ship's Side into the Stem.

Wind, needs no Explanation, unless we say, it is a Motion of the Air, enclining to some one Part of the Horizon, and by its various Changes giving Life to Navigation There are as many Winds as Points of the Compass, that is, Thirty

two,

two, tho' ſome will allow but of four Winds, which are North, South, Eaſt and Weſt, ſubdividing the others into Halfs, Quarters, and Half-Quarters

The Wind largeth, ſignifies, that it grows fair, and comes aft

To Wind a Ship; is to bring her Head about, either with the Boat, or with ſome Oars out of her Hawſe or Stern-Ports, if ſhe be a ſmall Ship

The Ship Winds up, is when ſhe comes to ride by her Anchor

How Winds the Ship, is a Queſtion they ask when under Sail, and ſignifies, upon what Point of the Compaſs does ſhe lie with her Head

To Wind the Boat, is only to turn the Boat's Head about

The Winding-Tackle, is this A great double Block, with three Sheevers in it, which is faſt ſeaz'd to the End of a ſmall Cable, brought about the Head of the Maſt, and ſo ſerves for a Pendant This has a Guy brought to it from the Fore-Maſt, and into the Block there is reev'd Hawſer, which is alſo reev'd through another double Block, having a Strap at the End of it, which Strap being put through the Eye of the Slings, is lock'd into it with a Fid, and ſo ſerves to hoiſe the Goods The Fall is reev'd into the Snatch-Block, and ſo brought to the Capſtain, for heaving of weighty Goods.

The Winding-Tackle-Blocks ; are Main-Double-Blocks, with three Sheevers in each of them, and are fast seaz'd to the End of a small Cable, which is brought about the Head of the Mast, as may be seen above, under *Winding-Tackle*

The Windlass , is a long Piece of Timber, having some six or eight Squares, and is plac'd from one Side of the Ship to the other, aloft close abaft the Stem, where the Cables come in. It is only us'd in small Ships among the *English*, but more among the *Dutch*, and the Reason of it is, because they go very slightly Mann'd and the Windlass does purchase much more than the Capstain, and with no Danger to the Men, for they heave about the Windlass with Handspecks ; that is, Wooden Leavers, commonly us'd in removing any Thing that is ponderous, which they put into the Holes made at either End of it, and tho' they cannot heave forwards, or any one should fail, yet the Windlass will pawl it self, and so avoid all Danger Whereas at the Capstain, if any fail, they may be thrown from the Capstain, and their Brains beaten out against the Ship's Side, if they weigh in a Sea-Gate But the Capstain does purchase faster, and therefore the *English*, who have Men enough for it, use that There is also a Windlass in the Head of the Boat, to weigh the Anchor by the Buoy-Rope.

Wind-

Wind-taught. Any Thing that holds Wind aloft, which may prejudice the Ship's ſailing or riding, is ſaid to be Wind-taught; as too much Rigging, high Ropes, and the like Alſo when, they ride in any great Streſs, they bring their Yards alongſt Ships, and ſtrike down the Top-Maſts, and the like, becauſe they hold Wind-taught, that is, they hold Wind ſtifly; for Taught is the ſame as Tight, or Stiff.

Windward; is the Side from whence the Wind comes, oppoſite to the Leeward, which is the Side the Wind blows upon: So any Thing that is on that Side the Ship from whence the Wind comes, is ſaid to be to Windward

A Windward-Tide, is when the Tide runs againſt the Wind, as a Leeward Tide is that which runs down with the Wind The former makes the roughest Water

With the Metal, is a Phraſe among Gunners, ſignifying, that a Piece lies Point-blank

Wood and Wood, ſignifies the letting in of two Timbers one into another, ſo cloſe, that the Wood of the one joins cloſe to the Wood of the other

A Worm; is a Winding-Iron put upon the End of a Staff, and is us'd to draw the Shot out of a Gun, if there be Occaſion

Worming; is the laying of a ſmall Rope or Line alongſt, betwixt the Strands of a Cable or Hawser, the Use of it being to help and strengthen the Cable or other Rope to which it is join'd The *Dutch* do this to new Ropes, and others to old ones almost decay'd.

To Would, or *Woulding*; is to bind Ropes about any Mast, Yard, or the like, to keep on a Fish, or to strengthen it; Sometimes, when the Whoodings give Way by the over-charging of the Bolt-sprit, they are fain to would to the Bows; which is done by passing a Cable through both Sides, and so bringing it in again, and twisting it together with Handspeeks as strong as may be No Mast or Yard is ever fish'd, but it is also woulded; and this is call'd, the Woulding of the Masts or Yards Also the Ropes which come from the Beak-Head over the Bolt-sprit, and lash it fast down from rising off the Pillow, are call'd, the Wouldings of the Boltsprit

Y

YArds; are long round Pieces of Timber, somewhat thicker in the Middle than at the Ends, and hang by the Middle a-cross the Masts. The Use of them, to bear the Sails which are made fast to, and hang down from them. The several Yards belonging to a Ship are, the Sprit-Sail-Yard, hanging over the Boltsprit, the Sprit-Sail-Top Sail-Yard, over that again The Fore-Yard, belong-

ing

ing to the Fore-Maſt; the Fore-Top-Sail-Yard, to the Fore-Top-Maſt; and the Fore-Topgallant-Yard, over that again at the Fore-Topgallant-Maſt: The Main-Yard, at the Main-Maſt, the Main-Top-Sail-Yard, at the Main-Top-Maſt; and the Main-Topgallant-Yard, over the laſt, at the Main-Topgallant-Maſt. The Mizzen-Yard, at the Mizzen-Maſt; and this is the only Yard which does not hang ſquare with the Maſt, but ſloaping up and down; the reſt having ſquare Sails, and this a triangular one The laſt is the Mizzen-Top-Sail-Yard, at the Mizzen-Top-Maſt; and this hangs ſquare, and has a ſquare Sail, like the reſt The Terms us'd about the Yards are, *Top the Yards*, that is, make them hang even. *Brace the Yard*, that is, traverſe aft the Yard-Arm, whoſe Brace is hal'd

A Yaw. When the Ship is not ſteer'd ſteady, but goes in and out with her Head, they ſay, *She Yaws* This hinders a Ship's Way very much; and therefore Men of War in Chace put the ableſt Men to the Helm, who can keep her ſteadieſt and eveneſt upon a Point, which is the Reſult of Care and Judgment

A Yoak. When the Sea is ſo rough that Men cannot govern the Helm with their Hands, then they ſeaze two Blocks to the Helm, on each Side, at the End, and reeving two Falls through them, like

like Gunners Tackles, bring them to the Ship's Sides; and so some being at one Tackle, and some at the other, they govern the Helm as they are directed There is another Way of doing it, by taking a double Turn about the End of the Helm with a single Rope, the Ends thereof being belay'd fast to the Ship's Sides; and by this they guide the Helm, tho' not so easily as the other Way, but either of these is call'd, *A Yoak to steer by.*

FINIS.

Lightning Source UK Ltd.
Milton Keynes UK
UKOW07f1826170915

258830UK00005B/107/P

9 780699 132879